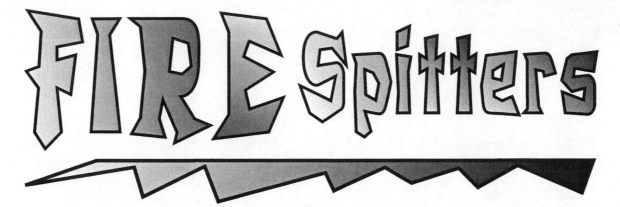

FIRE Spitters

**A Workbook
for Parents
(and others)
Who Want to
Successfully
Deal with a
Difficult and
Angry Child**

GARY BENTON, M.C.

Printed in Victoria, Canada.

Note for Librarians: a cataloguing record for this book that includes Dewey Classification and US Library of Congress numbers is available from the National Library of Canada. The complete cataloguing record can be obtained from the National Library's online database at:
www.nlc-bnc.ca/amicus/index-e.html
ISBN 1-4120-2044-1

GARY BENTON is well-known for the practical value
of his presentations at workshops and conferences. With over 20 years
of experience in working with young children, Gary knows what will
and will not work in dealing with difficult young students.

Gary is a frequent trainer and seminar presenter, providing programs on:
anger management, dealing with difficult children, building self-esteem
in children, communications skills, stress reduction, and team building.

Gary Benton, M.C.
gwbenton@aol.com

TRAFFORD

This book was published on-demand in cooperation with Trafford Publishing.
On-demand publishing is a unique process and service of making a book available for retail sale to the public taking advantage of on-demand manufacturing and Internet marketing. On-demand publishing includes promotions, retail sales, manufacturing, order fulfilment, accounting and collecting royalties on behalf of the author.
Suite 6E, 2333 Government St., Victoria, B.C. V8T 4P4, CANADA
Phone   250-383-6864   Toll-free 1-888-232-4444 (Canada & US)
Fax   250-383-6804   E-mail   sales@trafford.com
Web site www.trafford.com   TRAFFORD PUBLISHING IS A DIVISION OF TRAFFORD HOLDINGS LTD.
Trafford Catalogue #03-2623   www.trafford.com/robots/03-2623.html
10   9   8   7   6   5   4   3   2

For
Donna and Lindsey

Special thanks to Dr. Andrea Vangor, who got me started on this project;
to my uncle, John Benton, a successful writer on his own part, for helping me finish it;
and to the hundreds of men, women and children who shared some of the most
difficult moments of their lives with me and became my teachers.

CONTENTS

INTRODUCTION

I probably should start by explaining the title of this book. In my family we would describe someone as — "He was so mad he was spittin' fire!" So, Firespitters came to mean someone who is really, really angry.

I've learned a great deal about fire spitters over the years. As a family counselor and the director of a very large anger management program, I've worked with literally hundreds of fire spitters, from very young children to very old men. Some of the youngest fire spitters were only two or three. The oldest was eighty four. They were, of course, very different yet had some things in common. The most obvious thing they shared was how much their friends and family were tired of their anger. No one really wanted to be around these fire spitters when they were angry and so avoided doing things they thought might upset them. There was a great deal of avoiding. Not only did their family and friends avoid them but these individuals did a lot of avoiding, too. It seems no one is really happy when someone else is spitting fire, not even the fire spitter.

Even though this book is about dealing with difficult and angry children, some of you reading this are also fire spitters. Real, honest-to-goodness angry people who wish you weren't so angry. Good. This book will help you. The rest of you live with fire spitters and want things to be different. Good. This book is specifically designed to help you and them.

I should be honest and tell you I love angry people. They have so much energy and they want to solve problems so badly. What could be better? When I work with teachers I remind them that the angry child may not be the child in the most trouble in the classroom. It may be the isolated child, quiet and alone, who is really in trouble – the one nobody can reach emotionally. These are the ones who grow up to be dangerous. So long as angry children aren't isolated, there is a great deal of hope that they can become effective problem solvers as adults. And, after all, people are adults much longer than they are children. So we want to develop our children into successful adults. And, at the same time, we want them to be likable children who have reasonably rational adults in their lives. At least most of the time.

I want especially to thank two special fire spitters in my life: my brother, Mark, who was the first real fire spitter I have ever known, and my wife, Donna, a genuine fire spitter (from what her parents and sister tell me) from the get-go. I suppose it goes without saying that I love them both.

Mark, who is now a pastor, has grown into a wonderful man, a loving and responsible husband and father and a great uncle. He and his wife, amazingly, are raising their own fire spitter. "What goes around, comes around."

Donna, my wife of over 26 years as of this writing, has grown into a wonderful, beautiful, loving and responsible wife and mother. She runs her own business and is active in our church and in our daughter's school. And she had the good sense to marry me!

If you could have talked to their parents a number of years ago, you wouldn't have gotten much hope. These were challenging children. They were strong willed and, once their minds were made up to go a particular way, pity the person who tried to stop them. Truthfully, that hasn't changed much. They still are powerful, goal directed people.

How to go from raising a challenging and difficult child to a having a responsible and caring adult is the subject of this book. For Mark and Donna, their parents, teachers and mentors all had a hand in their eventual development. There are some keys that we will discuss, ways of keeping an angry and difficult child on the path to success. By the end of this book, I hope you find yourself appreciating the strength of character in your difficult child more often than you feel convinced there is no way to raise this child without one of you ending up on the funny farm.

CHAPTER 1

PUTTING ON THE OXYGEN MASK

I was flying to Los Angeles recently and, as usual, the flight attendant was going over the safety issues. Now, honestly, I've heard those instructions enough to not be very interested anymore; but, for whatever reason, I listened this time. Should the cabin lose air pressure, the flight attendant explained, an oxygen mask would fall out from the compartment above me and I was to put it on. I was assured that even though the little bag wouldn't fill up, oxygen would be flowing to the mask. She went on to say, "If you are traveling with a child or someone who may need assistance, *put the mask on yourself first, then help the other person with you.*"

There's an important lesson in that comment and we'll come to it soon. Meanwhile, I hope you'll find this book to be more than you expected. I hope you'll find it to be more work and more rewarding than any other thing you've done to improve yourself as a parent. I hope that someday your child thanks you for all the things you did to contribute to his or her success. And I hope this book will be a part of that experience.

For sure you won't find this a recipe book for getting good child behavior. There aren't any recipe books written exactly about you or your child. We both know that. Rather, this book is about what it takes for *you* to write the recipes for getting the behavior you want from your child (most of the time). Even so, I've always been bothered by the saying, "Children don't come with instructions." Because, actually, I believe that they do. The instructions are self contained in both the child and in his or her parents. I heard a very respected pediatrician speaking on a morning talk show giving advice to parents. He asked this question: "Do you know what a pediatrician is *really* worth?" The host said, "No." "Two grandmothers," he replied. "Two grandmothers know everything a pediatrician knows, and then some."

HOPE

You are your child's best and most enduring hope for the future. You will be there when the school sends him home sick. You will be there when she learns to ride her bike and falls and gets discouraged and hurt. You will be there when his favorite pet dies. You will be there when she experiences her first love and, soon after, no doubt, her first heartbreak. So it's not a teacher who will be there. Nor a counselor. Nor a pastor. It's you! And your child knows that and wants that and needs that.

I have worked with children and families as a therapist for more than 27 years now. Most of the children I've worked with and most of the families, too, for that matter, were in serious trouble. Many of the children had been abused, neglected, used. And yet in almost all cases the child longed to return home, back to the abusive mother or father, back to the family. There is something so powerful and so important about the parent-child bond that it transcends most of life's problems.

So this book will begin by focusing on you, then on your child, and finally on what the two of you can do together to solve most of the life problems that you now face and will confront again in the future. I'll start with you because I truly believe parents are the key people in a child's life, and that you will pay the price for your child's success long after everyone else in the world has given up. If you are like me, you are often bewildered by parents who will stick by their serial killer son believing in his innocence until the very end. I have often thought those parents lived in denial about the terrible crimes and immeasurable suffering their child has caused. Maybe they do. But, maybe, it's more than that. Maybe it's the way all of us as parents and children are really designed to be – bonded to each other forever.

So I'll begin with the most important person in a child's life: his or her parent. You. Once you've had a chance to work on "you," we will work on your child. A friend of mine says the secret to understanding is to ask the right questions. Hopefully you will be asking the right questions and discovering new answers as we work our way through the challenge of raising a difficult and angry child.

FREE ADVICE

This book will start with the flight attendant's advice. *Take care of yourself first* before you take care of this challenging child. Put on your *self control first*, before you try to control this difficult child. Be Internally Controlled. Not Externally Controlled.

Now admittedly that is easier said than done. However, it's the key to self control and to how that relates to controlling your child.

I heard Dr. James Dobson – Don't miss his book <u>The Strong Willed Child</u> – tell a story about a mother he'd worked with who had a 13 year old who was completely out of control. He asked her when she felt she'd lost control of this child, and she told him this story: when the boy was only three and as she put him into his crib for a nap, he spit into his mother's face As the story goes (and he tells it much better than I) she grew angrier and the child kept spitting, until finally the mother completely "lost it" – a scene that sounds very nearly abusive. As she left the room, the child spit on the door as she closed it.

In an anger management program I directed, I worked with a man who had been court- ordered to our program because he had beaten up his wife. When he described the incident, he explained that he had come home to find her in bed with his best friend. He chased the man out and then beat up his wife. When I asked him when he'd first noticed the relationship with his wife was going sour, he replied: "When I found her in bed with my best friend. Up to that point we had a great relationship."

Now for both of those folks the relationship was out of control much earlier than they had guessed. That poor mother had lost control long before her little boy was born. That poor man had lost control long before he'd even met his wife. What happened to them can happen to any of us. We can find ourselves believing that our happiness, our success, our peace of mind . . . are "out there" somewhere. We believe that those feelings somehow reside in our marriage, our job, our friends or even in our children. But if you believe your child's behavior points to your success as a parent, you may be facing the same fate as that poor mother who tried to reason with her three-year-old and nearly ended up abusing him. If you believe your happiness in relationships depends on how your loved ones act, you may face the same fate as that man who abused the woman he loved.

WHO OWNS YOU?

Here's an explanation of the theory (sometimes called "Locus of Control") I'm using. We have one of two choices in the world. We can choose to be **Internally** Controlled or **Externally** Controlled. People who are *Internally* controlled believe: "I make me feel, think and act." People who are *Externally* controlled believe: "Others make me feel, think and act." Your success and mine as a parent depend heavily upon which choice we make. If we believe our feelings are tied to our child's behavior or to other people's opinions about us or our child, we will be *Externally* controlled. We will find ourselves trying to please others or trying to change situations over which we have little or no control. From here the next step is to regard what others think as more important than what we, ourselves, think; and soon enough our child, or other people, or circumstances, will control our emotions.

Staying *Internally* controlled, however, means that we decide what to feel based on our own actions. Then even in the face of criticism we decide for ourselves whether we are doing as good a job of parenting as we can. If we are doing the best job we can, then – though others may not share our opinion – we can still feel good about ourselves. If our child is acting up (and we feel embarrassed) we can still feel good knowing we are doing what we can in the situation. No child is perfect. No parent makes all the right decisions. No situation guarantees our success. However, if we are Internally Controlled we are going to feel and be far more successful than if we are Externally Controlled. Someone once said, "Trying to please everyone is the surest way to failure."

It would be nice to say that we can make the choice and stick to it. However, most of us go back and forth between being Internally and Externally controlled. This book will help you learn to be Internally controlled (at least most of the time) and help you to help your child learn the same valuable lesson.

WHO OWNS YOUR FEELINGS?

You have to decide whether your child can make you angry or not. I contend *nobody* can make you (or me) feel angry. Or happy. Or sad. Or frustrated. Or any other feeling. Oh, I know, it's easy to live in a theoretical world and pretend that no one can make us "feel." I'm not really suggesting you won't feel good or bad based on how others act or treat you. However, I do claim that if you make a decision to *actively seek* to be internally controlled, you can change and control how you feel.

Here's an example: I have a friend who hates waiting in lines. He contends this is a leftover from his days in the military when he had to wait in lines everywhere. As you can imagine, he has a hard time enjoying himself at places like Disneyland. Even though the lines move right along, he still finds that the longer he has to wait the more impatient he becomes. I, on the other hand, have sort of a fondness for lines. I am a person who works with people. I find people absolutely fascinating. And lines are full of people. People to talk to, people to observe, people to learn from. For a "people person" a line is one long living story. (It's the same reason I can go to the mall shopping with my wife and daughter. I'm not much of a shopper but, boy, there are so many interesting people there!) So he and I can be standing together in line and he'll be feeling more and more frustrated while I'll be feeling more and more fascinated. We're both in the same line but our *interpretation* of the experience is very different. Thus our feelings about the experience are different. That's why it is sometimes so much easier to enjoy your children's screams of delight and laughter than a stranger's. Your kids are having fun, but their kids are disruptive, out of control, obnoxious. That's also why your child bursting out laughing in the back yard is so much less stressful than your child bursting out laughing in the middle of church. Same laughter, same child, but you'll have quite different interpretations and much different feelings.

Consider this example. Imagine you are having the worst day of your life. You get stuck in traffic on the way to an important appointment and get there late. While you're there you are treated terribly because you came late and feel foolish. On the way home you get a flat tire and it is pouring rain. Some crazy driver cuts you off in traffic and then makes a rude gesture as he drives by. You get home late, tired, hungry, mad and just wanting to get out of your wet clothes, curl up in front of the TV and vegetate. As you walk in the door the phone is ringing. You drop your stuff, race to get it and say "hello." The voice on the other end says, "Hi, this is the Publisher's Clearinghouse. Congratulations! You are our 10 Million Dollar Winner. We'd like to come over with a television crew and present you your first check of $167,000. Okay?"

Now, how long do suppose it would take you to change your feelings? An hour or two? Probably not. My guess is your feelings would change instantly. You see, we can only have one feeling at a time. All of our feelings belong to us. Thus we can pick whichever one we want and feel it whenever we choose.

Keep this example in mind when, in the next chapter, we talk about memory building.

SUCCESS OR FAILURE?

Being Externally controlled is a prescription for disaster. I have never met a successful person who was Externally controlled. Of the successful people I've met they are always aware of others and their needs, are often gracious, and know their own success is very much the result of the people around them. However, they never lose track of the idea that their own behavior determines how they define their success.

A friend of mine is a salesman. A very successful salesman. He defines his success by the number of calls he makes in a day, not by the number of sales. He says he subscribes to the "cheetah" theory of sales. He says a cheetah is not really a very efficient hunter. A cheetah is fast but doesn't have much endurance. Consequently, if the prey is hard to catch the cheetah will probably not eat. The beauty of the cheetah is that he keeps on trying. He hunts a lot, and now and then catches one. My friend claims it's the same with sales. Even if you're a lousy salesperson, if you make a lot of calls you'll get some results. So he doesn't feel he has a good deal of control over whether a person buys today or not. Maybe they have the money and maybe they don't. Maybe they'll buy next week. Maybe their child is sick and they are distracted and wouldn't take his product if it was free. He doesn't have any control over most of these variables. But he does control how many calls he makes and so that is what he focuses on.

I have never met a person with an anger management problem who *did not* have an External Locus of Control. Angry people really believe that if others would change, their own lives would get better. You'll often hear an angry person say, "If I had more money, I would be happier." Or, "If my child would act right, I wouldn't be so angry." Or, "If my boss wasn't such a tightwad, I would be better at work." Or any number of things. It's the belief that somehow, some way, the answer to one's life's problems are "out there" – somewhere in the control of others. Or it's just Fate. It's the same belief system that drives people to spend their hard-earned money on lotto tickets (although, those big jackpots are hard to pass up!) or to complain about their life or their clothes or house or car when they compare themselves to "the Joneses". It's the belief a parent has when he or she says in one's heart, "If my child was more like that one I'd be a good parent, too. Anyone can successfully raise an easy child. They ought to try raising my girl (or boy) and then they'd know how hard it is." Jealousy, too, invariably indicates a person who is Externally controlled.

THE FIRST STEP TO SUCCESS

You will be far more successful if you define your success as a parent based on your own behavior rather than on the behavior of your child. You can't really decide that *you* are successful because your child reads early or walks early or passes the math class or gets asked to the school prom. You should decide if you are successful based on what *you* have done or are doing that encourages the behavior you want.

I will use this example again when I talk about memory, but I'll tell you a personal story about me and my daughter. When Lindsey was in the first grade she brought home her first report card. It was an outstanding report card and I was very proud. Now, to be honest, I was not only proud of her – I was proud of myself as well. In fact I may have been more proud of myself than I was of her, since I believed then that she got good grades because I was such a wonderful father. As I was driving to work the next day I got to thinking about how great a father my daughter had but it also occurred to me that I had just decided to tie my self esteem as a father to how well my daughter does her homework. That worked fine in the first grade, but I knew (dreadfully) that junior high was coming (and it did, by the way). Tying my self esteem to my nice, successful first grader, was not such a great idea, I realized, since I knew she would be in eighth grade some day and that that could be a very different story. So I decided I'd better not tie my self esteem as a father to how well my child does in school. Instead I determined to tie my self esteem to how well I supported her in school. I knew children whose parents are involved in their school activities get better grades. So I made a commitment to helping my daughter with her homework (and to go to as many school activities as possible). I learned to feel good about myself as a father by doing the things that I knew would help my daughter succeed in school. However, if she doesn't succeed in school I'll know that I've done the best I could to help. School success, is, after all, tied to *her* behavior, not mine. I don't attend the classes. I don't do the homework. I don't take the tests. I don't have to figure out how to get along with her teachers and peers. That is all *her* work. My job is to support her every chance I get. That's how I measure my success in the school arena – not on her grades, but on my supporting behavior.

DO WHAT YOU CAN

A young man I had worked with in a group home moved back to his parent's house. A few weeks later he attempted suicide and his family called me to the hospital. He was in a coma and hooked up to life support systems. While I was there, I talked to his doctor. I asked the doctor his opinion of this young man's chances of living and he replied, "I don't think they are very good. We aren't getting much brain activity. *But we want to give him every chance we can to live.*" The young man died and I think often about doctors and how they can face life and death every day. This young man's physician figured out his role. He couldn't make the young man live. He could only do all he was able to do to give him the *chance* to live.

As a parent you can only do the best you can to help your child develop into a responsible adult. You can't make all of the child's decisions. You can't pick his or her friends. You can't protect them from every possible danger and pain. You can only do what you can do.

You must stay Internally Controlled. You must decide that you are the one who is in control of your thoughts, feelings and actions. Your child can't make you hit him or hug him. You decide what to do. Your child can't make you love her or be angry with her. You decide what to feel. Your child can't make you think sad thoughts or happy thoughts. You decide what to think.

The poor mother whose three year old spit at her as she walked out the door had decided before she walked into his room that he could make her feel successful or unsuccessful as a mother. She was Externally controlled. When she felt unsuccessful, she tried to change *him* and failed and continued to fail for at least the next ten years. When the man found his wife in bed he had already decided she could make him happy or unhappy. When he found her in bed with his friend, he tried to change *her* and failed. (By the way, she divorced him and married the friend).

Children spit and are defiant. Loved ones sometimes make terrible mistakes. However, parents are successful or unsuccessful people based on what *they* do, day in and day out, regardless of their child's behavior. Spouses are successful or unsucessful based on what *they* do, day in and day out, regardless of their mate's behavior.

This book is about dealing with the difficult and angry child. You may often feel it is an emergency, that you should be calling "Mayday, Mayday!" It may feel like a plane crash and that you need air. But you will only succeed if you put the oxygen mask of Internal Control on yourself, first, before you try to help your child.

So, write this on one of those wonderful "Post-It" notes and put it where you will see it everyday: *"I make me think, feel and act, every single time."* Change is always from the inside, out. If you develop and maintain this view of yourself as a parent, you'll find your behavior will soon begin to change, as well. And you will become more successful. And your children will wonder what you are up to.

One last story before we go on. I worked with a young, single mom who came in for counseling. She explained that she "ruled by volume," which meant that as her three young boys got more and more out of control, she would yell louder and louder. She hated that about herself because her mother also ruled by volume and she didn't want to be like her mother. So, she came to counseling to find better ways to control her sons.

We talked and I learned she was really a wonderful, loving – but overwhelmed – mother. Her boys were about three, five and seven-and-a-half. They were active boys whose father had a new girlfriend and who was mostly absent from their lives, leaving it to their mom to do all of the parenting. She felt she was losing control of their behavior, and her own, and had vowed she was not going to let the divorce ruin her children's' happiness. She had told her boys that she was going to see the counselor because she wasn't happy about how their family was going. Now the boys weren't sure just what "going to see a counselor" really meant, but they picked up from mom that this was very serious. And they were very curious.

So we developed a plan. I suggested to her that she not change her yelling at all. But, at dinner that night, to sit down with the boys and tell them, "I've talked to the counselor and he thinks it's okay if I yell at you sometimes. So I'm going to keep on yelling. *But you had better not ever make me whisper.*" Now her first born wanted to know just what would happen if they did make her whisper. Her brilliant answer was (in a low voice) "you don't want to find out." And she left it at that. Truthfully she didn't have a clue, either. She wasn't going to abuse them and she wasn't going to give them away. And based on our assessment, they were doing well in school, with their peers, and at their church. They followed her rules (as well as any young children could) and she liked each of them for their unique personalities and talents. Really, nothing was wrong except that she didn't like yelling at them and the feeling that came with being out of control.

That evening the boys were the boys and she started yelling. After a short time she realized she was yelling and began to lower her voice. As it got closer to a whisper, she heard her oldest son say, "Cut it out you guys. Mom's starting to whisper!" And they did!

She came in the next week only to report how well she was doing, and then I talked to her about six months later on the telephone. By then she told me that not only did she not yell so much but she didn't ever whisper, either. Besides, the boys had gotten older. They had attained more self control, and life had gone on. She laughed and said she thought she had come to counseling to learn how to control her boys but walked out having learned how to control herself. Smart woman. She learned the magic of Internal Control.

LOCUS OF CONTROL

EXERCISE 1

How do you define your success as a parent?

On this sheet list up to five ways you measure your success.

An easy way to do this assignment is to fill in the blank at the end of this statement:

"I know I am doing a good job with my child (or children) when _____ ."

1. _____
   _____
   _____
   _____

2. _____
   _____
   _____
   _____

3. _____
   _____
   _____
   _____

4. _____
   _____
   _____
   _____

5. _____
   _____
   _____
   _____

LOCUS OF CONTROL

EXERCISE 2

An Internally Controlled person is someone who is Self controlled.
An Externally Controlled person is someone who is controlled by Others.

How do you define your success as a parent?

On this sheet list up to five ways you measure your success.

An easy way to do this assignment is to fill in the blank at the end of this statement:
NOW USING "I" STATEMENTS.
"I know I am doing a good job with my child (or children) when _____ ."

1. _____
_____
_____
_____

2. _____
_____
_____
_____

3. _____
_____
_____
_____

4. _____
_____
_____
_____

5. _____
_____
_____
_____

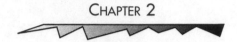

CHAPTER 2

WHAT DO ASPIRIN COMMERCIALS SELL?

Really. Have you asked yourself that? Some of the most interesting stuff on television are the commercials. The title of this chapter suggests one of my favorite questions to ask parent groups when I am speaking. You'll get a chance to figure this out pretty soon. I want you to just sit back and relax. I'll ask you to put the book down in a moment and do something you probably rarely do: watch TV. Specifically, I want you to watch commercials. As you do, answer this question: "What is this commercial selling?"

MEMORY BUILDING

Your conscious memory, my conscious memory, your child's conscious memory is built in two pieces: a factual piece and a feeling piece. In other words, we remember both facts and feelings. Research (and experience) tell us that facts with strong emotions or feelings attached to them are far more likely to be remembered than facts with little or no emotion attached to them. For example, many of us can remember many details about the birth of our children years ago but may have trouble remembering where we were just two weeks ago. The birth of a child has many strong emotions attached to it while our day two weeks ago, unless there was some remarkable experience, is hardly remembered at all.

On top of that, experiences repeated over a period of time are easier to remember than experiences we have just one time. Try to solve these math problems: 2X4 = ?; 3X5 = ?; 4X7 = ?; 9X6 = ?; 6X17 = ?. Did you suddenly stop doing these in your head, from memory, and have to figure out the last one on paper, or at least visualize it? Most people don't practice their times tables everyday but can remember, years and years later, the answers from 1X1 to 12X12. That's because you repeated the memorization over and over, possibly for weeks.

So, conscious memory is a combination of strong emotional experiences and/or repeated experiences.

HOMEWORK

Right now, go watch TV and figure out what *feeling* each commercial is selling. You might also notice whether you've ever seen that commercial before or heard it's music or jingle or catch phrase. The book will be here when you return.

Thank you. And the advertisers thank you, too. You are one of the few people in America who didn't get up and do something else when the commercial was playing.

My favorite example is aspirin commercials. You'll notice the first thing an aspirin commercial sells you is pain or stress. Before you see the product, before you hear how well it works or that it is "doctor recommended," before you see some graphic of it speeding relief to the area of pain, you will likely see an actor or actress who looks to be in terrible pain, telling you how much pain they are (or were) in until they took the product.

Aspirin commercials want you to think of their product when you feel a headache. So, they sell you the pain and tie their product to it. Beer commercials sell fun, romance, sex, friendship and status and tie their product to these things. They want you to think of their product when you want one of those feelings. Believe me, highly paid marketing experts work long hours to decide just exactly which feelings to tie to their products. It isn't by accident that pain is tied to aspirin, or romance to beer.

Basically commercials sell feelings and tie their products to those feelings so, when you have the feeling, you'll think of the product. Or, when you want the feeling, you'll think of the product. And they do it over and over. They get you both ways: with feelings and with repetition.

SELLING YOURSELF TO YOUR CHILD

As a parent, keep in mind that the feeling is left long after the facts have changed or are even forgotten. You'll probably notice it is easier to remember the feelings of a commercial than many of the specific details in it. You may also notice you have a feeling about a product when you see it in a store rather than remember many of the details of its commercials.

If you are like us, you have friends you haven't seen in years. Good friends, but you or they have moved away and you stay in touch with cards around the holidays or an occasional phone call or letter. My wife and I recently went to Boise on business and we have good friends there, Pam and Doug, whom we hadn't seen in at least six years. We weren't together ten minutes before it felt like we hadn't missed a beat in all that time. We laughed just as much, enjoyed each other just as much, caught up on old times and new adventures and vowed to see each other more often. Everything about Pam and Doug's life (not to mention my wife's and mine) had changed. New jobs, new houses, older children, new experiences, yet, among us the feelings of friendship and love hadn't changed at all. The feelings stay the same long after the facts have changed or been forgotten.

I read Stephen Covey's outstanding book, The 7 Habits of Highly Effective People (three times) and took it to heart to write a mission statement for my life. Well, to be honest, there is no way to write it for my whole life (although I did write a vision statement that, so far, seems fairly timeless.) Instead I wrote it for one year and now re-write it each year in December. I tried to organize it around the six major areas of responsibility in my life: family, finances, physical self, mental/educational self, Spiritual self and my social self.

A FEELING MISSION

In the family part of my life I am a father. One of my missions is to be my daughter's favorite teacher. I will never be her best teacher, especially in math. But I can make learning fun and positive when she is with me, so that is my goal. I don't worry, when we do homework together, about getting the right answers. The right answers are not that important to me. Now, to be clear, the right answers are important to

Lindsey and so they become important to me. But, for me, the goal is not simply to get the right answers. My goal is that we will like each other as much as, or better, at the end of the homework experience than we did at the beginning. I intend to laugh sometime during the homework and I intend for Lindsey to look me up when she needs help with her homework because it is a fun and a valuable experience for her.

Let me tell you why. I know what advertisers know: she will remember how it *felt* to do homework with her dad long after she has forgotten whether we got number 14 right or wrong. Homework is problem solving – a great life lesson. I want her to believe that she and her dad can solve problems together and like each other in the process. So the right answers are not as important to me as the feelings my daughter attaches to me. By staying Internally Controlled, I decide what feelings I want my daughter to attach to me and then do all I can to "sell" her those feelings. Being her favorite teacher means I have to be helpful, that we need to come up with mostly right answers. I have to be encouraging, to have faith in her abilities, to believe she can do it without me (since the idea of teaching is to send the students off into the world prepared to meet the challenges without the teacher). I have to be patient and kind, to have time available and, for her sake as well as mine, I need to be able to laugh at my own mistakes.

PICK A FEELING, ANY FEELING

What feelings do you want your children to attach to you? Do you want them to think of you as angry, impatient, tired, hurried, resentful? Probably not. Do you want your children to feel fear, guilt, anger, hate or resentment when they are around you? Probably not. You need to *decide* what feelings you want to set as your goal for your children to feel when they deal with you about anything, from the trivial to the important. This is the first and most important step to maintaining your sense of Internal Control as a parent.

I suggest you write down for yourself a list of the feelings you want your children to have every time they deal with you, whether this is when you are having fun together or when you are disciplining them. You and your children have thousands of experiences together ahead of you and most of them will be forgotten over time. But you can bet that your children will have feelings about you that will never be forgotten even if they can't remember how they ever learned to feel that way in the first place.

Here's a suggested list of feelings:

Love	Patience	Faithfulness
Joy	Kindness	Gentleness
Peace	Goodness	Self Control

Imagine how different your life would be if, every time you dealt with your children, they felt one or more of the feelings on this list. Imagine how different *you* would feel if you worked to communicate one of those feelings every time you dealt with your children (or anyone).

We began the book by talking about taking control of ourselves before we try to take Control of our children that is, by putting the oxygen mask of self control on ourselves before we put it on our child.

STEP ONE

The first step of that process is to *consciously decide* you are in control of your own feelings. You and I can decide and set a goal to make sure our children feel one of those nine feelings every time they come in contact with us. When we wake them up in the morning for school, we can show them both joy and gentleness. When they are struggling in their school or with friends, we can be faithful and loving. When they are doing the dishes or cleaning their room or telling us a story that is important to them, we can be patient. When they are in trouble and need to face the consequences of their behavior, we can be kind. When life is too hurried and overwhelming, we can be peaceful.

The key, of course, is for *you* to feel those feelings. As the book goes on we will talk about my ideas of how to find those feelings. But, for now, just do this one task: write down ONE of those feelings on three Post-It notes (the same feeling on each one) and put a note where you will see it the first thing in the morning (in my house the coffee pot is usually the first thing I actually, semi-consciously see), put another note in the first place you will see when you come home from work (the dashboard of your car could be a place) and the third one in a place you will see it each night before you go to bed (maybe the bathroom mirror). Now, if you can, also put a fourth note someplace where you are likely to see it during the day. Commit yourself to working on that feeling for the next three weeks (21 days) and, like the commercial advertisers, remind yourself to "sell" that feeling every time you deal with your children. If you really do this assignment, I promise your life will begin to change – first for the worse (since all children test to see if you really mean it) and then for the better (since it is hard to dislike a person who is actively trying to live with love, joy, peace, patience, kindness, goodness, gentleness, faithfulness and self control).

Truthfully, successfully dealing with a difficult and angry child means you *decide* you are in control of your life, even your feelings. If you are Internally Controlled and working to express one of those positive feelings, you'll find yourself acting very differently and, as a result, your children will respond very differently. You will be less concerned with controlling the child you feel is controlling you and more concerned with controlling yourself. The more *Internal self Control* you feel, the less *External Control* your child will have on you. With *Internal* Control comes success.

No one is perfect. No one can always be patient or always be kind or always be loving. However, by making a decision to do so, anyone can be patient more often than not, or kind more often than not, or loving more often than not. One good way to succeed is to tell your children exactly what you intend to do. Have you noticed how many companies have their mission statement right where their customers can see it? I was at a large variety store recently and they had it right at each checkstand where both I and the clerk could see it. Telling your children you will be patient with them for the next three weeks makes you instantly accountable and, interestingly, they will probably try to help you succeed. It's much more fun to be around a patient parent than an impatient one.

So, to quote Nike: "Just Do It" (what a great slogan!). Put this book someplace where you will find it in three weeks or so and we will go on from here.

CORE VALUES EXERCISE

Here is a list of words that represent many people's values. This list may not represent all of your personal core values so add any words that might not be on this list that you would like on yours.

Love	Joy	Peace	Kindness
Wealth	Power	Success	Learning
Happiness	Family	Faith	Honesty
Wisdom	Laughter	Equality	Respect
_____	_____	_____	_____
_____	_____	_____	_____

Now that you have listed your top core values, take a moment and narrow those down to just ten.

Did you find yourself making some trades?

Now, narrow your top ten to only five.

Did you find that was even more difficult?

Now, narrow your top five to just two.

That is even harder but you probably now are looking at the two values you really believe in and will believe in your whole life.

The tough question: Are you actively, purposely living and teaching these values to your child (or children) every day?

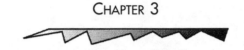

Chapter 3

"IF IT WAS EASY EVERYBODY'D DO IT."
— Jack Nicklaus on golf

Let's see. You haven't picked the book up now for at least three weeks! Oh, I know. What good is a book if it isn't being read? Still, I would prefer you take your time as you read this because, otherwise, the ideas and techniques will only be ideas and techniques, not new ways of taking on old problems. I assume you've heard this definition: *"Insanity is doing the same thing and expecting different results."* In the first chapter I asked you to take some time and practice Internal Control. In the second chapter I asked you to take three weeks and practice one of nine positive feelings so this would be linked to you in your child's mind. If you have simply read the book so far and said to yourself, "Hmmm, that's a good idea," but without applying the idea to your everyday life, you probably are doing the same things that led to your picking up this book in the first place. And getting the same results.

STRESS

As the director of a very large and active anger management program, I would get a call now and then from local radio and television people to get my comment on some act of violence in our community. Once I got a call from a radio station because a man had a rifle and was shooting at cars as they drove on one of our major freeways. It was a live interview and the reporter said, "Well, Mr. Benton, do you believe this man is angry and shooting at cars because of the high stress in our society?" I answered, "No. He's a nut. If you give a gun to a nut eventually they shoot at people." I didn't get many more calls from the radio station.

Good grief. There are thousands and thousands of people under extreme stress who don't go off and shoot at people. Stress doesn't cause anger. It does cause all kinds of physical problems and other problem-solving difficulties, as you'll see in this chapter. But it doesn't cause anger or violence.

This chapter and the next are about stress. As usual, we will start with you first. Then, in the next chapter, we will look at stress in your child.

Stress is common to all of us. It occurs as problems mount in our life. It's important to know stress is self-defined (as are problems) and what may be stressful for one person is not necessarily stressful for another. For example, soldiers on a battlefield report feeling no more stress than you and I do in our normal day to day activities.

My brother-in-law, Tony, lives in a rural part of the area near me. He reports feeling a great deal of stress driving into Seattle. I commute to Seattle often and most days would have a hard time noticing the stress of the traffic. On the other hand, Tony reports no stress driving from his home in western Washington, over the Cascade Mountains, through the rest of Washington, across Idaho, up the winding, two-lane highway to Glacier National Park in Montana, *towing a trailer*. I, on the other hand, find that *very* stressful. Especially towing the trailer. (I recently bought an old MG that didn't run and had to tow it home. I called Tony who not only towed it home but managed to back the car right into my garage. Thank goodness my sister-in-law, Darlene, had the good sense to marry him).

There are various lists of things most people find stressful and I'll share the one that seems most true for me. You, of course, are very likely to have a different list of top stresses, but see if some of these don't ring true.

THE USUAL CULPRITS

1. **MONEY**, how to get more, spend less or put some away. Interestingly, people who win big lottery jackpots report an *increase* in stress. Wouldn't you love to try on some of *that* stress someday?

2. **TIME**, including a lack of time for fun as a family, a lack of personal time, and too many things to fit into a day.

3. **CHILD DISCIPLINE OR BEHAVIOR,** including school problems; fights among siblings, and getting chores done in the family.

4. **TOO MANY RESPONSIBILITIES,** at home because people won't share in responsibilities or because our personal standards are too high, and at work where there are too many tasks to complete in a day.

5, **NOT ENOUGH "COUPLE TIME"** or poor communication and problem solving as a couple, poor sex life.

6. **GUILT** for not accomplishing more or planning better for the future.

7. **TELEVISION** because it often paints unrealistically good and bad pictures of life. (I know someone who only allows himself to watch one hour of TV news a week. He says more than that poisons his life.)

8. **NOISE,** particularly noise we can't control. Did you know the sound of a jackhammer is less stressful if you are the one operating it? Noise beyond our control raises our blood pressure, heart rate and anxiety. It may prevent sleep and can cause ear damage because the timpanic membrane in your ear is stiffened over a long period of time.

9. **CHRONIC INJURY OR ILLNESSES,** which can cause loss of sleep, frustration and hopelessness. It can also be a stress if you live with someone who has a chronic problem such as a back injury or a chronic illness such as diabetes or even alcoholism.

10. **IN-LAW TROUBLE,** enough said.

Do any of these sound like problems you might experience sometime this week? Parents of young children talk about meal and bed times as stressful (parents of teenagers talk about meal and bed times as stressful, too, but for different reasons).

HOW STRESS AFFECTS PARENTING

The problem with stress for parents is that it affects our *problem solving* ability. An interesting thing about people is that we actually problem solve *better* as our stress level increases slightly. If you've ever given an important speech or presentation you probably "psyched' yourself up some. It's common for athletes to "psyche up" before a game or for actors and actresses to "psyche up" before a performance. What we are trying to do in those cases is to raise our stress level some to improve our problem solving ability. And it often works.

As stress continues to mount in our life, however, our problem solving ability doesn't continue to increase. For a while, it doesn't decrease either. It just comes to an optimum point and stays there. So some stress may be good to help us solve problems, but more stress is not necessarily better.

As stress continues to mount, our problem solving ability starts to drop. As it does, often our stress increases and our problem solving ability drops faster, increasing our stress even more. If you've ever been so stressed out that you couldn't remember your phone number or where you put your glasses or shoes or purse, you know what I mean.

Often we see people who "hit the wall" with stress make really dumb decisions or act in ways not normal for them. They become more emotional, make poor problem-solving decisions, and they may try to escape by doing impulsive things to make themselves feel better (shop more, drink more, buy sailboats, have affairs).

FINDING THE FOUNTAIN OF YOUTH – AND REGRETTING IT

As parents "stress out" we find them "regressing." Regression merely means we go back to earlier problem-solving behavior: we get younger. Let me give you an example.

Ever since my daughter started school (about the third week of summer) she has run out of ideas to keep herself entertained. (I won't go into my opinion here of the idea of year around schools but, as a parent, it would have saved my sanity more than once.) So, my little girl, whom I dearly love, will walk up to me and declare, "I'm bored!" Now, it's not in some sweet, kind, patient voice. Oh no. She says it in this whiny, grating voice that goes right to the part of my brain that says I am somehow responsible for her entertainment. So, being a reasonable dad and feeling just a little stress, I begin to suggest ideas. Each one is met with her comments such as, "that's dumb" or "that's boring" or "I've already done that." By this time, I have to tell you, I'm moving right up against my stress wall; and a little voice is speaking in my head saying, "So help me, I have spent about 14 million dollars on toys for you – play with one of them!"

I should explain. I live in the Pacific Northwest. I don't believe in "channeling." However, I have driven past local celebrity J Z Knight's house (she supposedly channels a 30,000 year old warrior named Ramtha). If you can channel 30,000-year-old warriors, there is money to be made. What a place! Her fence is worth more than my house. However, I still don't believe in channeling.

That said, my stress will continue to increase and, soon enough, I will hit my stress wall. Lo and behold, I begin to channel. Now, I don't channel some warrior from past ages. Oh no, I channel my dad. All of a sudden his words enter my mind and his voice comes out of my mouth and I find myself saying to my daughter, "You're bored? You're bored!!? Well, I can put you to work! There's always work to do around here!" And off I go. Now, honestly, that usually doesn't help much. But, at that moment it's all I can think of – so I say it.

Regression means we go back to earlier problem-solving behavior, usually behavior we learned as a child. If you've ever found yourself saying something to your child that you remember your parent saying to you, you've experienced regression. You may also find, as I often do, that many of the things I learned as a child are very useful. Not everything we learned is bad and not everything our children are learning from us is bad, either. However, the key is to be sure that the things you want your children to learn as they grow up are the things you want to teach them; not things you suddenly find coming out of your mouth unexpectedly. In its own way this, too, is a form of External Control. Instead of *choosing* what we want our child to hear and learn, we give up our present control and allow ourselves to be controlled by our past.

A SAD FACT OF LIFE

Let me tell you a sad statistic, based on my experience and research in the domestic violence program I directed. The best predictor that a little boy will grow up to abuse his wife or girl friend is that he saw his mother get hit. The two best predictors that a little girl will grow up and fall in love with an abuser is that she saw her mother get hit and that she was sexually abused as a child. I can't tell you how many young men have sat in my office after being arrested for abusing their wives or girl friends who said "I don't know what happened – I just reacted." And when I asked them, they said, "Yes, my dad did hit my mom." I also could never count all the young women who have sat crying in my counseling office (trying to survive a relationship filled with domestic violence) who said, "Yes, I was sexually abused growing up and my mom was hit by my dad."

It is important that you handle your stress on an everyday basis. Your child is learning from you all the time. You can't tell how your tomorrow is going to go. You can do what you can today to get ready for tomorrow. It's the same message as the flight attendant told us in the first chapter: *"Put the mask on yourself first, then on your child."*

STEPS TO REDUCE STRESS

There are two steps to really reducing stress: *identify it* and practice *self care*. I have two assignments for you. The first will take a week (8 days) and probably would be better if you did it for a month. The second will take the rest of your life, but you'll do it in small doses.

I have seen people apply these two ideas to their lives with wonderful results. The key to success, of course, is to start. So, even though I'm sure it sounds over-whelming, especially if you already feel under stress, trust me, this will really help.

STRESS CHART

Use this chart to identify your personal stresses. **Today**, in the left hand column, write down everything you find stressful. (If you are going to name names, be wise. A loved one might see this and not like the idea of being called a stress in your life.) Don't ignore the weather, your job, traffic or illness (yours or a loved one's). You can refer back to the list I gave you near the beginning of this chapter for other ideas. **Tomorrow** and for the next 7 days, check off those things you experienced. Don't evaluate whether they were stressful or not. Just check off daily whether they were a part of your day.

STRESS	Mon.	Tues.	Wed.	Thurs.	Fri.	Sat.	Sun.
(EXAMPLE) Traffic	x	x	x	x	x		
(EXAMPLE) Pay bills				x	x		
•							
•							
•							
•							
•							
•							
•							
•							
•							
•							
•							
•							
•							
•							
•							
•							
•							

WHAT DID YOU LEARN?

You will probably notice two things: first, some days are more stressful than others. Second, as you begin to identify stresses in your life you'll add them to this list and it will be longer at the end of the week than it was at the beginning.

FIRST STEP

The first step to really getting on top of your stress is to *Identify* those things you find stressful. It's been said we don't feel stress about the things for which we are prepared; it's the unexpected things that cause the stress. So the more you can learn to expect, the less likely you are to be surprised and have stress added to your life.

Another valuable outcome of identifying your stresses is that you have a chance to control them *at their source*. It's another chance for you to exercise Internal Control and to avoid being Externally Controlled by your stresses. Stressful events happen, but you will be able to *choose* your responses better if you become more aware of the potential stresses.

For example, if you know the day before a holiday that the traffic home from work will be awful, you can plan to handle that stress. As I mentioned, I commute through downtown Seattle. On the day before a holiday I make sure I have a lot of tapes I enjoy in my car. Often, what is normally about an hour-long commute will turn into a two-and-a-half hour commute. If I've planned for that and if I've told my family I'll be late, it simply turns my car into a (slowly) rolling library. I'd rather be home, to be sure, but at least I'm not feeling much stress and I feel my time hasn't been totally wasted.

SECOND STEP

The second step is *Self Care*. There are tons of books written on stress reduction and self care. And most of them are really very good. You might also look for books about "burn out" because these, too, often deal with stress and taking care of yourself. However, ask around. There may be a book a friend has read that you'll find very valuable. As always, with any self help book, including this one, they work a lot better if you read and apply the knowledge. *"Knowledge is not power, applied knowledge is power."*

I, of course, have some suggestions about Self Care, too. And, if you are curious, yes, I do apply them to my life. And, no, I am not overweight (although the effects of gravity are working). And, yes, I am careful about fats in my diet (but largely because my wife is more committed to low fat than I am and has raised my consciousness). And, no, I don't regard myself as a health nut of any sort, nor do I run marathons (I played baseball growing up and never could figure out those track people who ran and ran to nowhere for no reason. Chasing a baseball made so much more sense.) And, yes, I do regard channel surfing as an aerobic exercise.

So, enough already.

I (and many others) break Self Care into five areas: Physical, Psychological, Social, Spiritual and Intellectual. The key to Self Care is balancing the five areas. You can *overdo* any of those areas and therefore *under* do the others. You'll probably also find that some areas are simply easier for you to pursue than others. But you will find that your stress will drop dramatically if you create a good Self Care plan and stick to it day after day. You'll also find that you just feel better about yourself, and your mood and outlook on life will improve.

1.   Physical Self Care is anything you do, *on purpose*, to improve your body. For example, walking, jogging, riding a bike, swimming, playing sports that require movement, stretching, eating smart, resting, sleeping all qualify as good for you physically. And, if you've ever watched exercise programs on television, "Always check with your doctor before starting any exercise program." Actually, just having an annual check up with your doctor is a great way to start taking care of yourself physically.

2.   Psychological Self Care is anything you do, *on purpose*, to understand yourself better. For example: reading this book counts, as does any self help book (if you apply it) – talking to a friend about important feelings and values, taking a class or workshop, keeping a journal, going for counseling, joining a self help group, going to church. The key is to live an "examined life" where you take time to look at yourself and to ask yourself if you are living as you know you should.

3.   Social Self Care is anything you do, *on purpose*, with others to improve your relationships. For example: going out to dinner or a movie with friends, playing team sports, going to work, being part of a service club or volunteer group, spending time with your family, caring for a pet, looking up an old friend, making a new one, being a part of any organized activity, *participating* in your faith.

4.   Spiritual Self Care is anything you do, *on purpose*, to gain a broader perspective on life and your core values. For example, volunteering to help others, traveling to other countries, traveling to the other side of town, attending your place of worship, reading Spiritual books, going out into nature, hiking, taking care of a garden, making or appreciating music, writing a mission statement for your life, learning about and giving your time or money to an important cause.

5.   Intellectual Self Care is anything you do, *on purpose*, to challenge your mind. For example: playing games, doing or putting together puzzles, reading books from other times or cultures, developing a consuming hobby, having stimulating discussions, doing or reading research, watching educational television, getting involved in politics, learning a new skill.

All of these Self Care areas require a commitment on your part. Again, the key is balance. You'll notice I emphasized "on purpose" for each of those. Self Care is only effective if we *consciously choose* to do it. It you find it "just happened" that, for example, your friend called you, enjoy it, but don't count it as a true Self Care activity. You need to live your life, *on purpose*, not by accident or chance.

YOUR SELF CARE PLAN

On this page list three Self Care activities *in each area* you will do over the next three weeks.

PHYSICAL

1 _____
2 _____
3 _____

PSYCHOLOGICAL

1 _____
2 _____
3 _____

SOCIAL

1 _____
2 _____
3 _____

SPIRITUAL

1 _____
2 _____
3 _____

INTELLECTUAL

1 _____
2 _____
3 _____

You need to commit about 20 minutes a day to Self Care activities. For good physical Self Care you should include about 100 minutes of aerobic activity a week. Feel free to combine areas, you could walk fast with a friend three mornings a week and get both social and physical Self Care accomplished. You can go to church and get social, spiritual and psychological Self Care accomplished in one morning (what a deal!)

On this page, write out your weekly calendar of Self Care activities. If you have a weekly plan and you goof up one day, it isn't a loss because you already have your plan for tomorrow in place.

SUNDAY: (Suggestion: go to church. You get three self care activities at once! Social, Spiritual and Psychological.)

_____

_____

MONDAY: (Suggestion: start the day with a brisk 20 to 30 minute walk.)

_____

_____

TUESDAY: (Suggestion: take a walk again and read a book, magazine or newspaper for 20 minutes or so, for pleasure.)

_____

_____

WEDNESDAY: (Suggestion: take another walk, write in your journal, call a friend)

_____

_____

THURSDAY: (Suggestion; take another walk, read that book again, volunteer somewhere for an hour)

_____

_____

FRIDAY: (Suggestion: take another walk (remember you are trying for 100 minutes of exercise). Get together with the friend you called Wednesday, sum up your week in your journal)

_____

_____

SATURDAY: (Suggestion: sleep in. Work in your yard or garden or take off and enjoy nature or people or whatever makes you smile and relax)

_____

_____

If you find yourself sad or low, this can really help: eat a banana, take a walk and go help someone less fortunate. Potassium and tryptophan, exercise and looking at the world from a different perspective, can make all the difference in your perspective on the world.

SOME SOBERING STATISTICS

50% of all good Self Care programs fail the first day. Here is the classic failure statement: *"I'll start tomorrow."*

Of those that start, 50% fail within the first three weeks. Usually there is a "crisis point" you must face and get through. If you decide to walk, one morning it will be raining. If you decide to read, one evening your family will demand all of your time. If you decide to attend a social function, your car will have a flat tire. It's the way life goes when we commit to change. A pastor friend of mine insists we should expect three battles every time we make a commitment to change for the better. If you win the three battles, the war is mostly over. *If you can keep going through the third week, your odds of success automatically quadruple!*

GOOD NEWS

More than 85% of Self Care programs that last 3 months or longer will maintain themselves for the rest of your life.

SO, THE KEYS TO SUCCESS

1. Start, NOW.
2. Keep going, for three weeks (21 days).
3. Don't quit; your life is getting better, and you know it.

To sum up, briefly. We are talking about putting on the oxygen mask of self control. If your stress goes up you are likely to start problem solving by reacting and acting out messages you got as a child, not as the parent you want to be. List your stresses and track them every day for at least a week. Add three new Self Care habits to each of the five areas and pursue them through thick and thin. Don't quit. Don't be discouraged. Don't worry because it is a battle to be successful. Nothing worth something comes without a price. If *you* pay the price, *you* get to reap the benefits and rewards (and so will your loved ones).

CHILDHOOD LEARNING EXERCISE

Sometimes it pays to remember what lessons you learned as a child so that you can be better prepared when something comes up in your family today. Some of the lessons learned in childhood are very useful and some are not so useful. For this exercise, remember what lesson you learned about each of these areas:

What did you learn growing up about:

MONEY? _____

LOVE? _____

HONESTY? _____

FAMILY? _____

HEALTH? _____

YOUR BODY? _____

DISCIPLINE? _____

SEX? _____

SCHOOL? _____

YOUR INTELLIGENCE? _____

SELF CARE? _____

CARING FOR OTHERS? _____

RELIGION? _____

THE GOVERNMENT? _____

FOREIGNERS? _____

BOOKS? _____

PETS? _____

CHILDREN? _____

PARENTS? _____

If other thoughts came up while you were doing that exercise, write about them here so you don't forget. They are important lessons to remember, whether good or bad.

CHAPTER 4

YOUR CHILD'S STRESS

Four-year-old Katie came to her preschool one day and seemed in no mood to be patient with anyone. During the day she pretty well refused much of what her teachers asked of her and once, during free time, she deliberately pushed over a class mate who then struck her head on a table. When I later consulted with the teachers about Katie they said she didn't seem to feel any sorrow or guilt about what she had done. "It's almost like she did it just to see what would happen. I don't think she was sorry at all that the little girl got hurt," her teacher elaborated.

If you had the time then to look at Katie's life in detail you'd have found many of the stresses you'll read about later in this chapter. Her parents were under financial stress, she was sensitive to certain foods, she had difficulty understanding how to relate to people; and, though she was big and quite verbal for her age, she was still quite emotionally immature.

Most likely, of course, no one has written a book about you or your family. Even this book, as much as I'd like it to be 100% useful to you and your family, won't really tell the story. Besides, you and your family are always growing and changing. New experiences are ahead of you every day, and each one will have a small (or occasionally large) impact on how life goes from that point on. So, especially in this chapter, read everything with a "grain of salt" and keep in mind I am talking about things that are *generally* true but *not always* true for every child or every parent.

Before we begin, lets start, as always, with you. You are now on your first week of Self Care. You are working on balance, you are exercising more, resting more, seeing your friends and family more, being more spiritually active, reading a book or two, enjoying educational television – just a whole bunch of positive changes! Congratulations. (Am I being a little too optimistic?) Then again, if you haven't exactly gotten into Self Care remember that wonderful Chinese proverb: "The journey of a thousand miles begins with one step." Just keep taking those steps.

The last chapter was about stress and how to reduce it in your life. This chapter is about your child's stress. As I've asked you to do over and over, put the oxygen mask on yourself first, then on your child. It's important for you to reduce your own stress so that you'll be better able to help your child reduce his or hers. As you will see, much of your child's anger is the direct result of an unmanageable amount of stress. The stress shows up in the form of behavior or attitudes. If you can figure out the *causes* of your child's stress, you can help him or her learn how to manage it. The first step is figuring out the *signs* of stress. However, dealing with the underlying *causes* of stress is the real key to success. So, this chapter is about your *child's* oxygen mask.

ONE OF THE BIG MYTHS

There is a tendency to believe that children don't feel stress, or not as much, anyway, as adults seem to feel. Did anyone ever tell you, "Enjoy your childhood. These are the best years of your life?" Someone usually told me that during a particularly bad day or time of my life. Maybe you had the same experience. I know that individual was trying to help, to let me (or you) see the "big picture" – but I found the advice just a little maddening. I still remember wishing I could be older so that I wouldn't have to go through whatever was the crisis of that moment. I really like my life at this age. In fact, I've enjoyed each age more than the previous one. Even if I could, I wouldn't go back and relive those "thrilling days of yesteryear." Would you? Really?

STRESS NUMBER ONE

There are some common stress producers for all children. One of the most common is "separation anxiety" which means the child is upset when his parents leave for awhile or, for some, when the parents merely leave the room. If you've ever dropped your child off at day care or a Sunday school class and the child was in tears and upset as you pushed him or her in the door, you have experienced separation anxiety. One theory is that young children don't have the same sense of time as adults and aren't sure, when you leave them, whether you are ever returning. I can remember being a rookie parent dropping my daughter off at her Sunday school class week after week and she'd be crying and carrying on, and my wife and I would be feeling terribly guilty. We would push her, as she resisted us, through the door of the class and leave as quickly as we could. Finally, my wife and I couldn't take it anymore. We went to apologize to the teacher for leaving our angry and difficult daughter with this unfortunate teacher. When we talked to Karen (a veteran Sunday school teacher with two and three year olds), she couldn't remember our daughter being unusually upset. In fact, she didn't really remember her crying and fussing much at all. So we told her how Lindsey would be crying as we pushed her into the class room and Karen, in her wisdom said, "Oh, that's just two year olds. They always stop when you (the parents) leave them and they get involved in other things in the class." What a relief! Our two year old was like all the other two year olds. And we weren't such terrible parents, after all.

"GOOD NIGHT, SLEEP TIGHT...."

You may also experience separation anxiety around bed time as your child is preparing to be left alone in his or her room with the door closed. In fact, you may find your child climbing into bed with you in the middle of the night, night after night.

I'm not anxious to open up a can of worms here but let me tell you a story of my daughter when she was old enough to crawl out of her bed and into ours.

IT'S 2 A.M. WHERE IS *YOUR* CHILD SLEEPING?

It was the middle of the night, of course, and I was sound asleep. Now, just why my daughter always crawled over *me* to get into our bed I'll never know, but she did. I think it's because I am much less likely to get angry in the middle of the night than my wife (Remember, she was a fire spitter), and Lindsey knew it. Anyway, this was one of those nights when she had come to crawl into bed with us and another of the many, many nights I would get up and put her back into her bed and tell her, "No, you can't sleep with us. You have to sleep in your own bed." This particular night I did the same thing and said the same thing and she replied, "You have somebody to sleep with!" Well, gosh, that's true. I didn't have to face being alone, in the dark, separated from someone I loved. I didn't have to deal with stress from separation anxiety.

There are lots of people who will give you advice about whether children should ever be allowed to sleep with their parents. You can hear everything from the "family bed" concept at one end of the spectrum to the idea that children should never be allowed to sleep with their parents because it starts a bad habit you may never be able to stop. (Let me tell you, when your child is 14 years old he or she wouldn't be caught dead in your bed, it's hard being in the same shopping mall with you). But I do think some children feel the separation anxiety more than others and, if you can tolerate it and still get some rest, a child snuggling up with one of his parents and falling asleep in their bed is not really so bad.

ONE HEALTHY RESPONSE

I was the director of an adoption agency. We placed children from, among other places, orphanages in Eastern Europe. It is not at all unusual for children who have been raised in orphanages to really need to spend a good deal of time bonding with their new parents. They have a very high sense of separation anxiety, often coupled with an attachment disorder. I was told by the experts, the ones who advise the parents with whom we place the orphans, that the worst thing a parent can do to a newly adopted child is have him or her sleep alone. The child isn't sure who will be there in the morning and may never have had any experience of living with the same adults for a whole day. For those children, any attempt they make to stay connected to their new parents is welcomed – even sleeping in their bed.

You may find your child wanting to sleep with you after a particularly traumatic experience. A child going through a divorce (remember Katie at the beginning of this chapter?) for example, may feel much better sleeping with his or her parent than alone. Every child and every circumstance and every parent is different. In this matter, follow your heart. Don't worry about what the experts say. You can always find one who agrees with you. I remember a cartoon I once saw: Two little "bag" ladies were talking and one was saying to the other, "The thing I love about psychiatrists is you can always find one who will testify in court that you're crazy."

"LIFE WITHOUT A DOG IS A MISTAKE" — SEEN ON A RUBBER STAMP

The best thing that ever happened for our daughter and her separation anxiety was our dog, Stella, who happily sleeps in her room (often on the bed, and, I know, some of you may be thinking "This guy is a nut; beside just letting the dog in the house, he even lets it sleep on his kid's bed!"). Still, for our daughter, it meant having someone she loves keeping her company, and dramatically reduced her anxiety over being alone.

DADS GET IT TOO

On the other hand, I also remember dropping my daughter off at her pre-school and, as she hopped out of the car and headed off to the class (without a look back at me), *I* felt some separation anxiety as I realized she was moving into her world and feeling pretty independent. If you've ever watched the movie, *Father of the Bride*, you've seen a father's separation anxiety with his adult daughter.

So, separation anxiety is a real source of stress for small children. The child doesn't know for sure you are ever coming back and wants to be bonded to you. As you realize your child is becoming more independent, that may also be a source of stress for you.

STRESS NUMBER TWO

There are a variety of other sources of stress as well. For young children, toilet training can be very stressful. This, too, is different for every child. If your child is struggling with this new skill, get a book about it at the library and follow the directions closely. You'll probably hear this advice:

1. **Be positive.** Reward the behavior you want to, but don't punish "accidents."
2. **Be sure your child is ready.** If he isn't sleeping dry through the night, probably you are asking too much of him.

3. Listen to your child. You may find she will tell you when she is ready for "big girl" underwear or she may make other such statements to indicate toilet training time is here. If you talk to veteran parents who have been through it more than once, you may well find that for one of their children toilet training was really easy while for another it was really difficult.

STRESS NUMBER THREE

For many children, new experiences are stressful. Starting school, moving, having a new baby in the family, having a new parent or parent figure in the family, new pets in the home, new foods and new routines – any or all of these can all produce stress. When we talk about discipline a little later in the book, I'll talk about one theory of brain organization that may help explain why this happens and how to prevent at least some of the discomfort.

STRESS NUMBER FOUR

Being disciplined is stressful (I've devoted a whole chapter later in this book to discipline). Any time a parent is angry with a child, there will be stress. Your child may need to be reassured that you will not abandon him when you are angry or when you put her into the "time out" place. To make matters even worse, as children become more independent (the "Terrible Two's" is the beginning of the development of independent thought and action), just taking orders can be stressful. So here we have your child who is in trouble, and you tell him or her to take a time out and we now have two stresses at the same time: being disciplined *and* taking orders. Don't be surprised if you get some resistance and some very real anger.

STRESS NUMBER FIVE

Learning to share is stressful. It seems sharing becomes an issue about the same time as the child develops the concept of "me" and "mine." For children to have a good self image and to learn to take care of themselves as adults, it's crucial that they learn to separate themselves from others and have a sense of selfishness. Unfortunately for us as parents (remember you and I have long since passed that developmental stage), having a selfish child is defined as bad. But I would encourage you to be very wise about this. A selfish young child is not the same as a selfish young adult. We all need to learn how to share, but not at the same time that we are learning we have control over our own lives, bodies, time, and possessions. Children who are allowed to be selfish when very young – and who learn they are masters of their own bodies and daily activities – will be less vulnerable as older children to people who would use or abuse them.

THE VALUE OF SELFISHNESS

You'll need to decide if you want to believe this or not, but let me share with you an idea about the value of allowing your child to be selfish, at least for a little while.

If you are like me, you want your child to grow up to be a caring and sharing person. Remember, we are not raising children – we are raising adults. Choosing to share is a moral decision made by people who know they have the choice to share or not. We cannot truly share what we don't believe we own. Learning, as a young child, that we own things – that some things are uniquely ours and that we can choose to give them or not – is an important step to developing the virtue of sharing what we have with those in need. I think you should always encourage your child to share but, at the same time, allow your young child to be selfish so as to learn to freely give later in life.

I have a friend who possessed very few things of his own while growing up and has since become very financially successful as an adult. He has no trouble sharing his wealth and, in fact, has done much good for many people because he knows it is his to freely give. He says that when he was small he refused to share anything, since he felt he had so little of his own. Now, however, he feels he has so much of his own that he can't wait to share it with those who are truly in need.

Sadly, however, he'd insist that his children always share and would get very upset and angry with them if they didn't. After all, they had so much (especially when he compared what his children had with what he had had as a child), that he insisted they never be selfish. Ironically, they have seemingly grown into selfish adults because they never really felt they had anything of their own. To this day they apparently don't feel a moral obligation to share because they were never allowed to be selfish when young.

STRESS NUMBER SIX, AND BEYOND

For you and your child, it is important that you have an idea of the kinds of things in his or her life that may be stressful. Here is a list of common stresses for children, in order of their impact. It is adapted from the "Social Readjustment Rating Scale" by Dr. Thomas H. Holmes.

Parent dies

Parents divorce

Parents separate

Parent travel as part of a job

Close family member dies

Personal injury or illness

Parent remarries

Parent fired from job

Parents reconcile

Mother goes to work

Change in the health of a family member (better or worse)

Mother becomes pregnant

School difficulties

Birth of a sibling

School readjustment (new teacher or class)

Change in family's financial situation (better or worse)

Injury or illness of a close friend

Starts a new (or changes) extracurricular activity (music lessons, Brownies, etc.)

Change in the number of fights with a sibling (more or less)

Threatened by violence at school

Theft of personal possessions

Changes in responsibilities at home

Older brother or sister leaves home

Trouble with grandparents

Outstanding personal achievement

Move to another city

Move to another part of town

Receives or loses a pet

Changes personal habits

Trouble with a teacher

Change in hours with baby sitter or day care center

Move to a new house

Changes to a new school

Changes play habits

Vacations with family

Changes friends

Attends summer camp

Changes sleeping habits

Change in the number of family get-togethers

Changes eating habits

Changes amount of TV viewing

Birthday party

Punished for not telling the truth

Whew! What an exhaustive list! It gives you an idea of all the different things, from the most stressful to the least stressful, that your child can experience. I noticed two glaring omissions (in my humble opinion). First, there was no mention of the parent's stress. Trust me, if you feel stressed about something, your child is going to feel stressed too. The second was being the victim of physical, sexual or emotional abuse. An abused child – or even one who is growing up in a family where someone is being abused – is under a great deal of stress and it is almost constant.

ANOTHER LIST

Here is a second list, again rated from the most to the least stressful, developed by Dr. Kaoru Yamamoto of Arizona State University. She asked fourth, fifth and sixth graders to rate events and she came up with this list, published in Self magazine, November, 1979.

Losing a parent

Going blind

Being held back in a grade

Wetting in class

Parental fights

Caught in a theft

Suspected of lying

A poor report card

Sent to the principal

Having an operation

Getting lost

Ridiculed in class

Moving to a new school

Scary dream

Not making 100 on a test or paper

Picked last on a team

Losing in a game

Going to the dentist

Giving a class report

New baby brother or sister

The experts expected a new baby sibling to be far more stressful for children than parents fighting, yet the opposite, from the children's point of view, was true. According to the research, settling problems in a family without fighting has a very positive impact on a child's well being and self esteem. You may have heard advice from experts that children should witness their parents fighting, otherwise they will grow up with a wrong sense of the way families "really" are and the way life and love "really" goes. I'm not sure that's good advice. I think children need to see their parents solve problems together but I don't think they need to be a witness to arguing and fighting. That will simply add to their stress and anxiety and will make your child's life more difficult.

HOMEWORK FOR YOU

This week I'd like you to use the lists from the previous pages as a guide and make a chart to track your child's stresses. Check off *each day* those experiences your child has that are considered stressful. This is the same assignment I asked you to do for yourself in the last chapter. The goal is to become more aware of your child's stresses. An important key to successful parenting is careful observation. By tracking your child's stressful experiences, you will probably begin to anticipate problems on some days more than others.

CHILD'S SOURCE OF STRESS LOG

STRESSFUL EVENT	Mon	Tues.	Wed	Thurs.	Fri.	Sat.	Sun.
(EXAMPLE) mom and dad argued			x		x		
(EXAMPLE) child was sick							x

TWO MORE STRESSES TO CONSIDER

Two stresses of children that we haven't talked about but that are very common and often overlooked are rest and diet. Parents need to be careful about both. If you did the assignment and found there were some problems that didn't seem to relate to any particular stress, it may be that something else is causing your child's difficult behavior. In that case, one good place to look for a source of stress is your child's basic biological needs – that means rest and diet. Remember, your child will do 90% of his or her growing in the first 18% of his or her life. If you are lucky, your child started out about 8 pounds. (If yours was a lot bigger when he or she started out, my condolences to the birth mother). Now he or she is already much bigger and will continue to grow. Growth takes plenty of energy and rest is essential to that process.

"A NAP, A NAP, MY KINGDOM FOR A NAP" – WITH APOLOGIES TO SHAKESPEARE

I realize that some children sleep easily and others not so easily. Our child was never much of a sleeper. She eliminated her morning nap by about age 8 months and her afternoon nap by about 16 months. Of course, all of our friends seemed to have children who would sleep most of the day and, boy, did we envy them. An active, non-sleeping toddler is not really a blessing, as some of you reading this book well know. However, we still insisted she go to her room and at least rest for awhile (partly for our own sanity, to be honest). The thing we did get, thankfully, was a child who could stay up but also sleep in. She was never one of those kids who could go to bed at midnight and still wake up at 6 am. We have friends with children who are going to get up early in the morning no matter when they go to bed (my parents had a kid like that too – me).

For our daughter, we didn't tell her she had to take a nap (which would start conflict). Instead, we told her she had to go to her room and play quietly. We called it "cruising" as in, "Lindsey, it's time for you to go to your room and cruise for a while." We would then take a nap when she was little. We needed the rest, too.

"OH PLEASE, TAKE JUST *ONE* BITE!?!"

Diet is the second area. I am not going to tell you how to feed your children. There is a whole industry full of experts on child nutrition, healthy eating habits, and food sensitivity. There are wonderful books written on this very subject. One of our early favorites was <u>Feed Me, I'm Yours</u> – still a very good resource book. I will tell you this, I have a friend, Dr. Andrea Vangor, who works with parents of children who are severely behaviorally disturbed, including children defined as autistic. She describes these children as having a "Social Understanding Deficit." In other words, they don't seem to be emotionally affected by adults and seem to show little emotional bonding to anyone. She thinks (and has very good scientific evidence to support this) that children can be far more sensitive to food than we think. She would suggest, if you have a child who exhibits hyperactivity, attention deficits or similar problems, feed your child foods that aren't likely to cause a negative behavioral reaction. Some foods that often cause behavior problems are: cow's milk (and it's products), wheat, corn, tomatoes, sugar, peanuts and strawberries. She will talk about the poor First Grade teacher with a hyperactive child in the room who was fed pizza the night before for dinner, had a big bowl of Fruit Loops with milk for breakfast and then wonders why the child can't sit still in class.

Her belief is that some children have a very hard time ignoring the stimulation in their bodies caused by food sensitivities or allergies. Now you can't just stop feeding your child milk, cheese, ice cream, toast, cereal, sugar, spaghetti, pizza, tomato sauce, or peanut butter with strawberry jam sandwiches. You have to substitute one form of nutrition with another that gives your child the same nutrition. It really pays to consult an expert on this before you make any changes. However, you may find as many parents have, especially with a difficult and angry child, that the food change alone makes a huge positive difference in the child's behavior.

SHE, AND HALF OF AMERICA

Another Lindsey story. Lindsey is allergic to cow's milk. When she has milk she gets a little bit hyperactive and very giddy. It's almost like she's been drinking alcohol. She laughs easily, has a hard time concentrating and gets just plain goofy for a while. Her ears itch, she often gets very red cheeks and she will make a number of what we called "random noises", sounds that don't mean anything or serve any purpose except to drive us crazy. When she was little it was much more obvious. Now that she's older she can tolerate more milk, but she still has to be careful. Of course, she loves milk, ice cream, cheese and pizza. Once we were out to eat at a restaurant and the waitress asked her what she wanted to drink with her meal. Lindsey turned to us and asked "can I have a glass of milk?" We both, together, said, "No, drink pop or juice or something else." I wish I could explain the look on the waitress's face as she watched these parents say "No" to milk and "Yes" to pop ("soda" for those of you east of the Rockies).

THE SIGNS OF STRESS LOG

Here is a little chart I got from a pre-school in my area. They use this to track what might be going on with a child who's having a behavior problem. You'll notice there are only three problem causes: food, rest, other. To use the chart, teachers and aides first try to briefly describe the incident that seemed to start the behavior (event). Then they ask themselves (and sometimes the child):

1) What the child most recently ate (food),

2) Did the Event occur just before or just after a time for a nap (rest),

3) Is there some known stress in the child's life (other).

You might try using this chart or something similar with your child for a few days. Perhaps a pattern will emerge that you can learn to help your child avoid in the future.

SIGNS OF STRESS LOG

STUDENT: _____ DATE: _____

	EVENT	FOOD	REST	OTHER
DAY 1				
DAY 2				
DAY 3				
DAY 4				
DAY 5				

MORE HOMEWORK

Boy, you are finding yourself with a bunch of homework this week! Remember, this is the beginning of changing how your firespitter acts and how you react. This is the good stuff we are adding to the foundation we spent building in the first three chapters.

We will focus on observing, charting and learning this week and, next week, look at some stress reducers for your child. Keep in mind, you know most of this already. The value of writing it down is that it helps you remember the patterns and when to look for the behavior you want to prevent.

THE HARD PART

For me, as a parent, one of the most difficult things to remember is that the signs of stress my child shows with negative attitudes or behavior are not the problem. It might help if you think about signs of stress the same way you think about red spots that indicate your child has chicken pox. The red spots are not the problem. They are simply the signs of the problem. If you spend all of your time trying to cover up or get rid of the red spots, you'll never get around to treating the real problem which is the virus that is causing the disease. In the same way, if you spend all of your time and energy trying to stop the behaviors that your child uses to show you they are feeling stress, you'll never get around to helping your child deal with the underlying *sources* of the stress.

The reason I want you to keep the chart is it will help you identify the *signs* that your child is feeling stress and, from that, you can look for and help your child either handle or eliminate the *sources* of the stress.

BEHAVIORS THAT MAY INDICATE YOUR CHILD IS EXPERIENCING STRESS:

Here are some behaviors to look for to decide if your child might be feeling some stress. I'll try to lay this out by age but keep in mind that all people develop differently; and what may be true for most four year olds may better fit your three year old. Or, if your child is like mine, kind of a slow developer (she didn't even have teeth until she was one), you may find what's true for two year olds is more accurate for your three year old. Here I have used "he" and "she" alternately. If you have a boy, read everything "he", if you have a girl, read everything "she."

AT TWO YEARS:

VERY NEGATIVE ATTITUDE. She won't take any orders. He won't cooperate. She won't play with peers. He seems to refuse to do anything.

OVERDOES EVERYTHING. He gets too angry, too happy, too sad, too possessive. She has tantrums quickly or may hit or bite. He is too afraid of new things, new people, dogs, noises or changes.

WON'T PLAY WITH OTHERS. He refuses to share anything. She would rather play with her old toys or "security object" like a blanket or doll. He won't consider going near a new child or stranger.

OLD PROBLEMS COME BACK. He won't take his nap. She won't go to bed without conflict. He begins to wet the bed. She wets her pants during the day. He is afraid of the dark. She refuses to eat certain foods she has eaten in the past.

AT THREE YEARS:

STARTS ACTING YOUNGER. He seems to act "babyish." She has temper tantrums. He is very jealous. She is very possessive of her toys or parents. He gets very bossy.

STARTS MAKING THINGS UP. She begins to tell "white lies." He seems to confuse fantasy and reality. She develops an imaginary playmate who is blamed for her behavior.

SPEECH GETS MORE DIFFICULT. She talks more baby talk. He begins to stutter. She begins to mispronounce or stumble over words. He begins to ask "Why?" about everything.

GETS UPSET EASILY. She gets angry easily. He is easily frustrated. She gets more destructive. He destroys his own or other's possessions.

GETS MORE ACTIVE. He seems to never stop moving. She seems to never stop talking. He refuses to take a nap. She refuses to go to bed. He stubbornly continues doing what he is asked to stop doing. She stubbornly refuses to do as she is told. He forgets to get to the toilet on time. She forgets to eat.

AT FOUR YEARS:

DEVELOPS NERVOUS HABITS. She blinks her eyes too much. He bites his nails. She sucks her thumb. He picks his nose. She must bring something from home to pre-school.

GETS MORE ACTIVE. He gets silly. She gets more rambunctious. He loves running, jumping, bouncing and slamming. She overdoes rhyming, mimicking or uses "bathroom" language.

EMBARRASSES ADULTS MORE EASILY. He exaggerates and boasts. She is overly interested in body parts and functions. He takes off his clothes and runs nude through the neighborhood. She tells stories of her parents' embarrassing behavior. He is excessive about seeking attention.

DEMONSTRATES MORE FEAR. He is afraid of the dark. She is afraid of dogs or cats. He is afraid of imagined things in his closet. She is afraid of a story or book, of a familiar friend or relative. He is afraid of things adults think are scary such as snakes, strangers, spiders or mice.

AT FIVE YEARS:

SEEKS MORE APPROVAL. He "shows off' to get his parent's approval. She tattles on others. He seeks praise from adults. She is upset if her parents don't approve of her work, art, notes or stories. He uses name calling to make himself more important.

ACTS YOUNGER. He slips into "baby talk." She acts more like a three year old than a five year old. He worries more. She develops irrational fears. He delays doing work. She puts off tasks. He has trouble adjusting to kindergarten.

AT SIX YEARS:

ACTIVITY LEVEL INCREASES. He has trouble sitting still in school. She has trouble being quiet in school. He spills more often. She bumps into things more often. He gets more aggressive. She throws more temper tantrums. He wants to be first. She wants to be best.

SOCIAL SKILLS GET WORSE. He is more sensitive to teasing. She is more shy. He is more jealous. She gets involved in peer and sibling rivalry. He has trouble making decisions. She complains about too many expectations from adults.

FEARS INCREASE. He is afraid of getting lost. She is afraid of making a mistake with her friends. He is afraid to speak up in school. She is afraid to talk to the teacher.

AT SEVEN YEARS:

MOODS BEGIN TO SHOW. He is more moody. She is more unhappy. He is easily saddened. She is more thoughtful.

SOCIAL SKILLS ARE AFFECTED. He seeks approval from parents. She seeks approval from peers. He is more selective about friends. She is more modest and seeks privacy in the bathroom or when dressing. He wants order and routine and gets upset when his life is disrupted or a sibling messes up his room. She begins to have models or media idols.

Now, remember, the "he" and "she" can be interchanged. Some behaviors I've listed are entirely normal and only become a source of concern when they happen too often or seem to appear suddenly.

DON'T IGNORE IT

For all children, increased fear and unusual behavior need to be addressed. You can't afford to ignore behavior and hope it will go away. The negative behavior is a *symptom* of what is going on with your child, *not the problem*. It merely is your child's way of showing that he or she has a problem that needs to be solved. As I keep emphasizing, the behavior is like the red spots of chicken pox. They are important indicators of a problem but not necessarily the problem itself. If you drop everything and only deal with the difficult behavior or attitude you may miss the opportunity to find the source of the stress. The *signs* of stress are not the *sources* of stress, just as the signs of a disease are not the sources of the disease.

For example, I know a little girl who was under severe stress because her parents were constantly fighting. One day she deliberately walked up to a school mate on the playground and simply hit her. If you decided this little girl was angry with the school mate and that was the source of her stress, you would have been mistaken. In fact, the *source* of her stress was at home although the *sign* of her stress showed up on the school playground.

For now, for this week, just track your child's behavior for signs of stress. Use that "Signs of Stress Log" I borrowed from my pre-school friends and make notes to yourself daily about your child. You may find some days are actually very nice while others seem full of problems from morning to night. On the tough days, try to figure out whether your child's diet or sleep or stress pattern has changed. Maybe it's a combination of things and they all add up to make a tough day for your child.

THE FEARS STORY

When Lindsey was five, she had a very difficult year. In October of that year my grandfather (her great-grandfather) died. She and he were very close and she had spent a good deal of time with him and her great grandmother. In December we sold and moved out of our house. It was the only home she had ever known and she lived across the street from her best friend at the time. We moved into an apartment and we couldn't keep our dog, Sam. In fact, Sam went to live with our now widowed grandmother so that she wouldn't be alone. We moved into a different school district and sent her to a different kindergarten. She rode the bus to school for the first time. If you would like to, go back to the two lists of stressful events from earlier in the chapter and imagine all the stresses that were loaded onto Lindsey at this time in her life.

In her school they were teaching the students about the dangers of smoking cigarettes. They explained how smoking could cause cancer. It was all part of a health program the school was teaching. Unfortunately for Lindsey, this was the last straw. One fateful morning she was on the bus on the way to kindergarten. Her new best friend got on the same bus a couple of stops after Lindsey. Her friend had been taken to the bus stop by her dad and they were waiting in his car for the bus. As Lindsey watched, her friend kissed her dad good-bye, hopped out of the car and headed for the bus. Lindsey looked back and saw him light up a cigarette. At that moment Lindsey decided, since her friend's dad smoked, if her friend touched Lindsey, she would get cancer and die. So, as her friend bounced into the bus and headed for the seat next to Lindsey, our frightened daughter shrunk back as far away from her friend as she could. When she got to school she told the teacher she had a stomach ache and was sent to the nurse where she stayed until it was time to go home. Over time her fear of smoking got bigger and bigger and bigger.

Keep in mind she is an only child. Being an only child she had many choices she wouldn't have had if there was a brother or sister in her life. She had the whole back seat of the car to herself. She didn't have to share her room with anyone. She didn't share her clothes or chair or anything else with a brother or sister.

Lindsey developed all kinds of "rules" to try to control this fear. She had the "smoke side" of the car and the "clean side" of the car. She had "smoke" clothes and "clean" clothes. She had the "smoke" side of her bed and the "clean" side of her bed. She had "smoke" pajamas and "clean" pajamas. It about drove us crazy. And what could we do? How do you explain cancer to a five year old?

A TRULY LOUSY DAD

One night I was sitting on her bed reading to her, as I often did. The story was done and it was time for bed and I began to tickle her. (We still have tickle fights). Anyway, I pushed her (unknowingly) onto the "smoke" side of the bed while she had on her "clean" pajamas and she burst into tears. I was fed up. I blew up and said, "I'm sick of all these smoke rules, go to bed!!" And I slammed out the door.

Well, I don't really want to be a lousy father. At that moment I was, however. I cooled down and went back in to apologize and Lindsey said, with tears in her eyes, "Daddy, when are my fears ever going to go away?" At that moment I realized she was as unable to control her fear as I was. We were both helpless.

So, I said, "Well honey, you know I am a counselor and I've been talking to my friends who have talked to lots of kids with fears (and I really had) and they said, when you are about six, your fears will just go away. You'll realize one day you just haven't thought about them much and they will be gone." Lindsey was about six weeks away from her sixth birthday at that time. Now, to be honest, my counselor friends had said, "All kids go through that and they just grow out of it when the stress reduces." But I knew that my little girl needed more specific answers and, most importantly, hope.

As parents our goal cannot be to eliminate all sources of stress in our child's life. As much as we'd love to, we can't prevent death, illness and all the disruptions of life. Keeping our children in a stress-free cocoon won't prepare them well for adult life. However, we can help reduce our child's stresses to a manageable load and teach him or her ways to cope with the stresses in life that can't be avoided.

Remember helping your child learn to walk? You probably helped him some with balance but, now and then, let him try it on his own. If she fell and got hurt, you comforted her. If he walked across the room, you cheered.

That's really all we are talking about now. Just as you looked for signs that your child was ready to walk and then helped him as he learned that complicated skill, so, too, I would encourage you to look for signs of stress and help your child develop the skills and balance necessary to successfully walk down that path.

When your child is struggling with stresses and its effects on his life, keep in mind that he, too, needs *hope*. He needs to know the stress won't last forever, that the trouble won't last forever, that the problem won't last forever. What does need to last forever is your love for him and your commitment to just hang in there until the next part of life begins.

So, put on your oxygen mask first. (I wish I had put mine on *before* I slammed out of Lindsey's room). Then, as we will explore in the next chapter, put the mask on your child. Give him or her an awareness that the two of you are in this together and the hope that the two of you will find the answer.

YOUR CHILD'S SIGNS OF STRESS
EXERCISE

For this exercise, observe your child and make a short note telling what happened. Then ask yourself if there might have been a stress that caused the behavior. Do this exercise for 7 days to see if you find a pattern.

EXP:	**Event**	**Food eaten?**	**Rest?**	**Me?**	**Other?**
Mon.	*Bit his brother*	*cereal & milk*	*nap okay*	*I'm okay*	*new puppy*

	Event	**Food eaten?**	**Rest?**	**Me?**	**Other?**
Mon.					
Mon.					
Mon.					
Tues.					
Tues.					
Tues.					
Wed.					
Wed.					
Wed.					
Thurs.					
Thurs.					
Thurs.					
Fri.					
Fri.					
Fri.					
Sat.					
Sat.					
Sat.					
Sun.					
Sun.					
Sun.					

You'll notice there are up to three observations to make each day. Keep it brief. You are looking for patterns and sources of stress.

CHAPTER 5

FINALLY, THE OXYGEN MASK FOR YOUR CHILD

Are you a part of a group somewhere? Perhaps you belong to a club or a choir. Do you remember being part of a team growing up? A member of the Boy Scouts or Blue Birds? Do you remember being rejected by a team or club or group? Perhaps you were cut from a team or not given a part in a school play or musical production.

This chapter is about reducing your child's stress by helping him or her meet the needs you and I have met by being a part of a group or club or team.

By now you are practicing Internal Control. You have a Feeling Goal for each of your children (probably you've written feeling words on Post-It notes all over the place). You are practicing stress reduction and have an active, effective Self Care program. You are observing the sign and sources of stress in your child's life, how your child demonstrates stress and you also recognize the most obvious stress producers in your child's life. You have put the oxygen mask on yourself first, so now it's time to go to work on your child's.

This chapter and the next will lay the foundation for reducing your child's stress and for making problem solving more successful. I'll refer back to this chapter and the next when we talk later about dealing with anger and discipline, so you might want to dog-ear these pages.

THE FOUR BASIC PSYCHOLOGICAL NEEDS:

I'll start by talking about four psychological needs we all have which are particularly crucial to the development of your child's emotional well-being. Understanding these four critical psychological needs is also the first step in *preventing* anger and difficult behavior.

Now, before starting. I should warn you that if you are successful at meeting the four basic psychological needs in your child, your son or daughter might not turn out exactly as you planned. As parents we tend to view our children as if they will never be anything but that – *children*. After all, so far that's the only way that we know them. However, remember, we parents are not raising a child – we are raising an adult. What this means is that being a successful child is not nearly as important as being a successful adult. I remember reading a study of the people who were at the top of their professions and businesses. In most cases, they were not the A students. They were the B and C students. As a parent I sometimes lose perspective about the really important skills and talents of my daughter in the quest for better grades or more cooperation or whatever I think, at the moment, will make her a better child. Hopefully you will use this chapter to look at your child – and at your relationship with him or her – just a little differently.

The other part of the commitment is that I will deal with her to help her become the best adult she can be, even if she doesn't particularly like my solution.

The Four Basic Psychological Needs are:

1. BELONGING
2. POWER
3. FREEDOM
4. FUN

THE FIRST NEED: BELONGING

The first and most important psychological need is *Belonging*. It's exactly what you're thinking: being part of the family. Being emotionally bonded to our parents and siblings. Being able to be identified as a part of your grandparents' heritage.

In our work with orphans and children who have been neglected, the Belonging need is the one most challenged. Orphans grow up not really "belonging" (or bonding) to parents. As a result, when they are adopted they often have a hard time trusting that an adult will be consistent in their lives. Sometimes these children are identified as having an "attachment disorder" and may have one of two curious behaviors: some will "attach" to everyone, almost as though any adult could be their parent. A young child might run to the arms of any person, even strangers, as easily as they run to their adoptive parents. Other children don't seem to attach to anyone. They don't want to be held and cuddled by their adoptive parents, they don't seem to show any distress when their parents leave, and they don't seem to care if their siblings are around or not.

Belonging is the most important need people have. You need to belong to the important people and groups in your life and your child needs to belong to the important people and groups in his life.

If you can, remember your first week at your most recent job. I'm willing to bet you went home at the end of each day that first week just worn out. I am also willing to bet, if there was a staff meeting that first week, you went to it, introduced yourself and barely said another word. Over time your job probably got more stressful, you added responsibilities, it got more complicated and you worked harder than that first week. Yet you probably went home each day about as tired as any other day and much less tired than each day that first week. The reason you were so tired and so reluctant to share your opinions was because you were working on your Belonging need at work. You were trying to fit in. You paid attention to how people dressed, where they parked their cars, when they went to lunch, whether they came to work on time or early or late, whether they went home on time or early or late, what you could talk to your boss about and what you couldn't, which co-worker you could laugh with and which one you could complain to, and a host of other things. All of those are the Belonging questions. You worked to be accepted by your co-workers and to fit into the group.

SOME IDEAS HOW TO MEET YOUR CHILD'S BELONGING NEEDS

When your child was born, she, too, needed to belong. If you got your child through marriage or adoption when she was a little older, you really need to work on helping your child belong. Every child needs to feel in her heart, "My parent and I are in this thing together." No matter what the "thing" is, your child needs to know that you are standing beside them. That's partly why I don't worry too much about the child who crawls into your bed in the middle of the night because she heard a noise or had a bad dream. She is learning an important lesson: "When things are bad, my mom or my dad is there for me." She is also demonstrating that she believes she belongs to you. So, even though it's a hassle, and you don't get much rest, and you think this will last forever, be thankful you have forged a bond with your child. That is the first step to long-term problem solving.

No matter how your child came into your life (birth, adoption, marriage, foster parenting), *always begin with Belonging*. You need to let them know, as soon as possible, "We are in this thing called life together, forever, like it or not."

MY FATHER'S THUMBS

My daughter and I have the same thumbs. Our thumbs, when we hold them up straight, bend sort of backward at the top knuckle. My wife's thumbs don't. Now and then I remind my daughter she belongs to me because we have the same thumbs. It's a joke, a playful part of the many running jokes we have between us. In fact I sing her a song that's a take off from Amy Grant's wonderful song, "My Father's Eyes," except I sing "She has her father's thumbs..." If I could sing, it would be even more effective, but it gets my daughter to roll her eyes and giggle – so it works.

Find the things you have in common with your children. Notice your eyes, or shape of your face, or if you can roll your tongue or have a bending thumb. It doesn't matter what it is. What is important is that you belong to each other. If your child is adopted or a step child, you can still find the things you have in common. What are your shared experiences? Play a "Do you remember the time we...?" game where you find something the two of you did together. Get out the photo album, the baby book, ride a bike together, care for a pet, conspire to grow a garden, play a joke on someone else together.

THE QUICKEST FIRST STEP TO MEETING THE BELONGING NEED

The belonging need is often met *visually*. If your child walks into the room, *always* look him in the eye. Never miss that opportunity. If you combine it with a smile and a hug, you will be miles ahead. People decide they belong with us when we look at them. That's why customer service people emphasize eye contact. Have you ever walked into a room and someone in the room didn't look at you? Do you remember how you felt? Most of us suddenly feel awkward if other's don't look at us when we enter a room. It's almost as if we are intruding. Well, as you can imagine, if your child enters the room and you don't look there is a subtle message: "You don't belong here." With an angry and difficult child, you'll find that doesn't help.

ONE QUICK REMEDY SUGGESTION

So, there you are, slaving over a hot stove. Dinner isn't going well. You're tired. You're hungry. You feel hassled. Then your child comes zipping into the kitchen making all kinds of noise and demanding your attention. What do you do? Take a deep breath, put on your oxygen mask first. Then turn, look right at him, smile, give him a hug and say: "I'll be with you in awhile; the dinner is going to go up in flames if I stop right now."

Now, admittedly, depending on what is for dinner, your child may *want* dinner to go up in flames. But I think you'll find, especially if you do this fairly consistently, your child will get the clue that this is not a good time to interrupt you *and* still get the message that she Belongs to you. When we talk about the next basic need, Power, I'll add a suggestion. The worst thing you can do is *not* look because you will give the message: "You don't belong here" – creating problems later that you want to avoid.

THE SECOND PSYCHOLOGICAL NEED: POWER

The next need is *Power*. Sometimes "Power" is a word that frightens people, probably because we tend to confuse it with *control,* which is not the same thing. Power is *influence.* Everyone needs to be important in the group or family of which we are a part. We want our opinions to count, to be heard when we speak, to be valued as an important member. In the business world, adults report the greatest frustration on the job when they feel they are not *heard* by their bosses and co-workers. In my work as a marriage and family therapist, the most frustrating problem reported by most couples and families is the inability to communicate. Men, women and children complained that they didn't feel heard or they believed their feelings and opinions were not important to their loved ones.

Often, parents of difficult and angry children feel powerless. You may feel you have little or no influence on your child and you may feel quite controlled by *them*. So you try to increase your power and control over them and then you find yourself involved in a huge power struggle. In a power struggle in a family, no matter who wins – everybody loses.

MEETING YOUR CHILD'S POWER NEED

Power needs are most often met by simply *listening*. I know, that sounds too simple. And, I know, you believe you already listen plenty to your child. And, I know, your child, if he or she gets your attention, will talk your ear off. Still, if you practice listening, really listening without interrupting or explaining, you will find you are going to have far more influence on your child than you thought possible. Nothing ever changes over night. You'll have to keep listening, long after you think you've listened enough. But, if your child believes you will listen to his side of the story (not necessarily agree with it), you'll find problem solving gets easier and easier.

A MARK STORY

My brother, Mark, who was a difficult child, taught me this lesson. He knows how hard it is to listen to a difficult child, especially when he has done something and now you're mad. *You* want to *tell* him what to do and how to act. You want to *tell* him how you feel. You want to *tell* him to stop his acting up. You don't feel particularly patient and in a listening mood.

But *that's the time to listen*. One of the commitments I made to my daughter when she was little is that I would always listen to her side of the story first. Now, I haven't always done that, as she can tell you. But I have done it more often than not and now, as a teenager, she knows I will ask her to tell her version of the story before I tell mine. And, you know what? There is *always* another side to every story. And now and then her side makes more sense than my side. And I have changed my mind more than once, and I've learned how to be fair. On the other hand, when I am right there are always consequences. That's only fair, too

EVER BEEN RED-FACED, SPUTTERING MAD? GOOD!

As I said, *Power is influence.* Your child is going to have influence with you if she is attached to you. In my opinion, one of the best things to build a child's self esteem is to be able to turn her normally calm, relaxed parent into a red-faced, angry parent. This may sound crazy but, for a moment at least, think about this: if you can't make your parents angry, you are obviously not a powerful person, no matter what you might do in the world. Honest. I worked with a young man who had two psychiatrists for parents and they were so clinical in their approach to him that no matter what he did they were forever analyzing and understanding his behavior and he couldn't make them mad. So he escalated his behavior more and more and eventually wound up arrested and placed in my group home. And his parents still didn't get angry. Even though he could have, he never moved back home because he finally found foster-parents he could influence. He didn't want to leave his foster-parents who he believed really cared about him, to return to his natural parents who, he believed, didn't care about him. The only difference was that his foster parents got mad when he did something wrong and he knew he was important to them.

A SUBTLE CONTRADICTION

Remember when I told you no one can make you feel anything you don't choose to feel? Well, ignore that for a moment. It is okay if your child "makes" you angry. Or happy. Or sad. Or proud. Our children need to be able to influence us emotionally. The power in relationships is the ability to affect another person. It is also the gateway to creativity. That's why close friends can often accomplish things together that they might never accomplish apart. That's why we hear so much about teamwork and why more and more companies are using retreats to build their teams before they try to take on big projects or create long range plans. That's also why we have so much more fun when we are in love and why we can spend hours together doing little things with great joy. Power. We are easily influenced by our loved one.

THE SECOND PART OF THE QUICK REMEDY

So, back to the kitchen where dinner could go up in flames as you stop to deal with your child. *Step one* is to look right at him, give him a smile and a hug, tell him dinner will go up in flames if you stop right now. That helps meet the **Belonging** need.

Step two is to give him something to do that will help you. Something that, if he does it, will make you smile and if he doesn't will make you disappointed and frown. Something that visibly shows that your child has Power in your life, that he can influence your feelings and behavior. Like set the table, hand you something you need from the counter or refrigerator, put a dish in the sink, anything within your child's ability. That helps meet the **Power** need.

So, here he comes, demanding your attention. You turn, look him in the eye, smile, hug, tell him you can't stop because dinner will go up in flames and then say: "I'm so glad you came in, I need some help with that dish. Can you hand it to me?"

HOW TO PRAISE

Let's talk for a minute about praise. Nearly every family and child therapist will tell you to praise behavior, not the person. Easier said than done but let me try to explain the techniques.

If your child does something, whether it's good or bad, *talk about how the behavior affects you*. For example, you ask your child to hand you the dish, and he does. Don't say, "Thank you, what a good boy you are for handing me the dish." You have praised the person (good boy). Instead say, "Thank you, I would have dropped that dish if I'd picked it up because my hands are slippery. You made my life much easier." You have praised the behavior and talked about its *effect* ("made my life much easier") on you. Now your boy can walk away and feel powerful. He had a positive influence in your life. Later, when we talk about discipline I'll come back to that same rule: always talk about how your child's behavior affects *you* before you launch into discipline. In fact, as often as you can, talk about how your child's behavior, good or bad, affects you. One of the most important lessons a children can learn is that his or her behavior affects others. This lesson is the basis for our morals, the development of our conscience and, eventually, our successful or unsuccessful relationships. Adult sociopaths and psychopaths (people who commit appalling crimes with no apparent remorse or guilt) appear to have little or no understanding of how their behavior affects others and consequently make their moral decisions based entirely on their own wants and needs.

The first two basic needs are Belonging and Power. Once those are met, we can go on to the third basic need.

THE THIRD NEED: FREEDOM

Freedom means having "unencumbered" choices. We feel free if we have a variety of choices in life and less free with fewer choices. For example, people in the United States often complain about taxes. Huge industries are dedicated to trying to avoid paying taxes. As I write this a "flat tax" idea is being kicked around in the media and is getting a great deal of support from Americans. Taxes are one of the few things in America about which we have little choice, and it is a source of irritation. Freedom is a powerful need for us all.

ORANGES, APPLES, BANANAS, PEARS (and more where that came from)

I was in Los Angeles waiting at an airport recently and talked to a young taxi driver who had moved here from a small country, formerly a part of the Soviet Union. He talked about how much he enjoyed America and complained, like all of us, about high gas prices and taxes. He also told me how much he loved the freedom in America. He told me the story of his grandmother who came to America just two months earlier. He and his family picked her up at the airport and, on the way home, stopped at their local grocery store to pick up a few things. His grandmother got into the produce section of the grocery store and started to cry. She had never seen so much fresh fruit and produce in her life.

If you want three oranges and have three hundred from which to choose, you will experience Freedom. If you want three oranges and the person behind the counter has one orange and, if you're lucky, a pear and that's what they hand you, like it or not, you will not feel much Freedom.

So, too, your child. If she feels she has no choice in important matters, if she experiences little Freedom, you'll find yourself with an angry child.

ONE FINGER TOUCH RULE

Let me tell you a story to illustrate. All children, especially toddlers, go through a developmental stage where they learn a great deal by touching and handling things. If your child has recently passed that stage, you'll remember it. If your child is in that stage, you know what I mean. Well, Lindsey, my daughter, went through that stage, too. She wanted to pick up everything she could reach and would go to great lengths to get her little hands on things. We would go to people's homes and spend half our time trying to keep her hands off things that looked expensive or fragile. When we would go to stores, one of us would shop and the other of us would hover around our daughter to prevent her from touching or picking up things we didn't want her to touch. I tended to be the hovering parent most often. Not only did it about drive me crazy, Lindsey would be prevented from touching something she wanted and then throw these loud, angry, very public tantrums. So we developed the "one finger touch" rule. The rule was, she could touch anything so long as she only used one finger. It worked for all three of us.

Now, I have to admit, it was not an instant success. Sometimes she would forget to touch with only one finger and sometimes I wouldn't let her touch something with any fingers and we would fuss at each other. But, generally, she was very good about it and it got us through a time when we could have been fighting over who was going to be the boss of whom. All my wife and I did was increase her freedom. She needed to touch things and we found a way that worked for both of us: she could touch and we could allow it, so long as it was with one finger.

Lindsey is now eighteen and enjoys a reasonable amount of Freedom. For example, she will go shopping at the mall with a friend to take care of her own shopping errands. She will be home a couple of hours later and we will never think about what she has touched or picked up. She has all the same freedoms in the mall any responsible person would have.

CHOICES, CHOICES

Your child needs to experience as many choices as is reasonable for his age. His job in life is to gradually expand his choices until, as an adult, he has all the choices anyone has. Your job, as a parent, is to limit his choices by your common sense. At three, Lindsey couldn't be trusted with easily breakable things. So we limited how she could experience those things and tried to give her as much freedom as we could. Fifteen years later, we don't limit her at all about what to touch or pick up, so she limits herself and rarely picks up easily breakable things just for the sake of picking them up.

You and your child can have a lot of fun meeting the Freedom need. You can offer all kinds of choices. Would you like to wear this shirt or that one to school today? Would you like to go to bed at 8, 8:15 or 8:30 tonight? Would you like to set the table or pick up the dishes at dinner? Would you like to play inside or out in the yard? Just think of the hundreds of choices you make for your child each week and give him a few of them. Not only does his sense of Freedom increase, but his ability to be a problem-solver later in life also increases because he will learn that problem-solving is easier if there is more than one choice.

THE FOURTH BASIC NEEDS: FUN

The final basic psychological need is Fun. Now, fun is fun. *It is always self-defined.* What you think of as fun and what I think of as fun may be very different but we both know it when we see it. Your family also knows what is fun. The key to having fun is to find it in the every day things in life, not just to manufacture it or save it only for the weekends or vacations or special events. You can have fun washing the dishes or folding the laundry or bathing the dog. You can have fun playing games in the car as you drive or waiting for the bus to pick you up.

TWO EXAMPLES

When Lindsey was very small I owned a green Opel Kadett station wagon. I bought it for very little money (which is about all I had at the time) and, except for the engine and a few vital accessories, most of it didn't work very well. Specifically the heater didn't work, the battery box bottom had rusted out so water leaked into the car when it rained, the brakes were thrilling (to say the least) to apply and the wagon faced some other challenges, too. It ran, however, quite dependably, and so, at that time of my life, I was very thankful. I would take Lindsey to her grandmother's house in that old car and we would play games. One of our favorites was "I'm thinking of something..." and we'd give a clue like "red and round." The other person would then have to guess what it was. The drive was about a half an hour and we'd play and talk and sing. Even though I sold it long ago and replaced it with cars with everything working, to this day, that is my daughter's favorite car.

At this moment my wife and daughter are in the living room by the fire (it's a Saturday). Donna is reading a book about raising teen age daughters while Lindsey is doing her homework. Even our dog is part of the party. (Now that I think about it, *I'm* the only one not in there. About time to quit writing for a while, I think.) Anyway, Donna is reading selected parts from the book and discussing it with Lindsey. They are having fun. In fact, now and then, there are gales of laughter floating down the hall where I am in my office at the computer. Fun is fun.

THE BEST INDICATOR OF A HEALTHY FAMILY

The most important thing for parents to realize is that fun is crucial to a healthy family and a healthy relationship. In fact, if the fun begins to go out of a relationship, the rest of the basic needs will begin to slip, too.

Ask yourself: How much do we laugh? What are the every day fun things we have in common? Can we laugh at ourselves? Do we smile when we see each other? Do we have fun as a family or is it more fun to be apart? Do we need to go away for fun or can we have it at home, too?

When Lindsey was very little, still in diapers, my wife would let her run around naked a few minutes before she gave her a bath. Lindsey would run, and squeal with delight and laugh and Donna would laugh and say: "She's celebrating her body!"

Do you remember when your child was just born and what a wonder it was to watch them move and grow and make sounds? It is an honest-to-goodness miracle that all that stuff, fingers and toes and ears and eyes and lungs and everything else, works together; not to mention that, in time, your child figured out how to make all of it work to his advantage. Bodies should be celebrated. It is fun that we can yell, or frown, or dance, or say funny words, or draw funny things.

FIND A REASON, EVERY DAY

Find a reason to laugh with your child every day. Even if you have to make a small fool of yourself, find the fun in it. Figure out how to make the mundane tasks more fun. Tell "when I was your age" stories when you fold the laundry or do the dishes. Play guessing games as you drive. Sing along with the radio. Get kids' tapes at the library and sing along or listen to them as you go. Make up stories or jokes or legends about the drivers around you.

To meet all four Basic Psychological Needs, especially if you think your relationship with your child is under some stress or is in trouble, begin with the first one, Belonging, and then add the others in order: Power, then Freedom, and then Fun. Many times parents make the mistake of trying to work from the last need, Fun, to the first, Belonging, and find at the end that there isn't much fun and that all their efforts were failures.

Instead, begin at the beginning and look at your child and assure him, "We are in this thing together." All the messages that reinforce how your child belongs to you are important. It's crucial that you *never* give the message, "I wish I didn't have you" or "I wish you were different." Sometimes parents will compare their children to others and say, "Why can't you be more like him?" That is a devastating message for a child and one that threatens his most important psychological need because, what the *child* hears you say is, "I wish *that* child belonged to me *instead* of you." Being compared to a brother or sister is even worse because the message your child hears is, "I wish I'd only had her and not you."

Take the time to establish Belonging first and then add Power. "Tell me your side of the story." Listen carefully and quietly to your child as you let her influence you. Tell him how you feel about him and his behavior. Ask her how she feels about *your* behavior. Let him influence you emotionally.

Add the third psychological need, Freedom, only when you are confident your child feels she belongs to you and has influenced you. Now you are ready to begin problem solving. Explore as many options as you and your child can think of together and settle on at least two choices you feel are good ones. Then give your child the choice.

Finally have Fun. Find fun wherever you can. Go away to find it or look for it under the beds at home. Find it in the sink or laundry basket or at the local park. Look for it all the time and learn what your child thinks is fun and try to do at least some of it with him.

If you spend your time and energy trying to help your child meet her basic psychological needs, you will find you have helped your child develop inner strengths and security. You will reduce the sources of stress in his life and equip him to deal with stresses that can't be avoided. In that process you'll find that from the very start you have prevented a great deal of your child's anger and difficult behavior.

YOU'VE GOT 'EM, TOO

Let me finish by reminding you that you, too, have the same basic needs. You, too, need to Belong. If you have ever been through a divorce or painful breakup, one of the most devastating messages you got was "I wish I'd never met you," or something similar. And it came from a person who, at one point in time, you had committed your love and life to. It is very painful to find that your Belonging need will not be met. So, to meet this need in your own life, be a part of a group or family that wants you around. Join a club or volunteer your talents. *Belong* somewhere, especially with your own family.

Allow yourself to be Powerful somewhere. Have influence. Be important. There are a many ways to be influential. I direct a non-profit counseling agency. People who donate their money or time to us are influential because we know and they know they have committed something of importance to us and our work. You can help in a service club, give time to your church, get involved in your child's school or just take cookies to a struggling neighbor and you will meet your power needs in a positive way. Nothing influences others as much as kindly commitment to their well being.

I wrote the first draft of this chapter just after the terrible bombing had taken place in Oklahoma City. On the news that day was a little story of a grade-school class that collected new washcloths and got them wet, put them in plastic bags and gave them to the rescuers who are digging out the victims of the blast. You can bet many of those washcloths went home with those rescuers and will never, ever be thrown away because of the kind commitment they represent. Those children in that class experienced Power in its best form. And you can, too.

Expand your Freedom. You can experience Freedom and increased choices by simply learning a new skill or taking a class in something you don't know. I took a cooking class last year at our local school (I am not a great chef but I like to try things out) and it was wonderful. Set goals and pursue them. Improve your body through exercise, or meet a new friend. The more choices you have, the more Freedom you will feel. One of the difficult realities of aging is that our choices gradually get more and more limited. If we live long enough, our life at the end is often not much different than our life at the beginning, perhaps getting to the point of being fed, bathed and clothed by others. Anger in young people who have few choices and anger in old people who have few choices is not really very different. Expand your choices and your life will get better.

Finally, you, too, need to have Fun. You know what you like and I know you can think of a hundred reasons to not do what you really want to do. I know you have time and money constraints. I know you worry what others might think if you do something too different. But, goodness, you only have one life. This isn't a rehearsal.

ONE LAST SUGGESTION

Review you Self Care list and see how the ideas you have written down meet your four basic psychological needs. Remember that balance is important and you need to do at least one thing in each category on your Self Care list every week.

Everyone needs times for rest and renewal, to regain perspective and develop a sense of gratitude for our life and our blessings. If you meet your own basic psychological needs and help your child meet hers, you will find you both will develop a sense of wonder and delight about the world and a sense of humor about yourselves, your successes and even your failures.

I think of former President Jimmy Carter who has chosen to invest his considerable talent, wisdom and energy in Habitat For Humanity. He builds houses for poor working people so they can move themselves and their families onto the road of home ownership and success. He is arguably one of the most intelligent Presidents of the twentieth century and could easily be treated like royalty on the lecture circuit. Instead he carries lumber and pounds nails, working on a solution he believes in. If you could talk to him I'd bet he'd tell you all of his psychological needs are being met, perhaps better now than at any other time in his life. He Belongs to an organization and a group of people. He has Power and is a person of influence, not only in the organization but also in the lives of the families each home benefits. He has Freedom because he is in a creative, problem solving process. He has Fun and, when interviewed, tells reporters what a great time he is having.

You and your child can experience this, in small doses, too. It's up to you to follow through and help yourself and your child meet the basic needs.

MEETING THE BASIC PSYCHOLOGICAL NEEDS
EXERCISE — Part 1

Here is an exercise to help you meet the Four Basic Psychological Needs with your child or children. Remember, always start with Belonging and then do the others in order, from the top down.

BELONGING: Look at and touch your child at all the "transition" times of the day (whenever you have been apart for awhile and are seeing each other again or you are about to part for a while). Put a check beside each time you meet this need:

____   first thing in the morning

____   before going to school or day care

____   before a nap

____   after the nap

____   after school ends

____   after playing outside or away from you

____   before dinner

____   after the dishes are done

____   before bedtime

____   any other time you have been apart for awhile

POWER: This need is met by listening. We listen with our ears and our bodies. Check off each time you listen:

____   I listened to my child and told him/her what he/she said.

____   I listened to my child and told him/her what he/she said.

____   I listened to my child and told him/her what he/she said.

____   I listened to my child and told him/her what he/she said.

____   I matched my child's body language when he/she talked.

____   I matched my child's body language when he/she talked.

____   I matched my child's body language when he/she talked.

____   I matched my child's body language when he/she talked.

MEETING THE BASIC PSYCHOLOGICAL NEEDS
EXERCISE — Part 2

FREEDOM: The need to have *choices*. Check off each time you gave your child a choice:

____   I let my child choose his/her own breakfast
____   I let my child choose his/her own clothes
____   I let my child choose his/her own snacks
____   I let my child choose his/her own chore to do
____   I let my child choose his/her own (reasonable) bed time
____   I let my child choose his/her own toys to play with
____   I let my child choose his/her own book to read
____   I let my child choose his/her own way to make me smile
____   I let my child choose his/her own way to spend free time

FUN: The need to be spontaneous, to laugh, to let off steam, to relax and be creative. Write down each time you and your child had fun or laughed.

We had fun this way: _____

We had fun this way: _____

We had fun this way: _____

We had fun this way: _____

We had fun this way: _____

We had fun this way: _____

MEETING MY OWN BASIC PSYCHOLOGICAL NEEDS
EXERCISE

As a parent, it is just as important for you to meet your Basic Psychological Needs as it is for your child. In fact, if you are good at meeting your needs you will be modeling for your child how he or she can meet his or her needs, especially as an adult. Remember the exercise you did about the things you learned in your family? What lessons do you want your child or children to learn from growing up in your family?

BELONGING: Write down in this space the things you do to belong to a group and your family. Who looks at you? Who touches you? Who do you look at? Who do you touch?

_____

_____

_____

_____

_____

_____

_____

POWER: Write down in this space the things you do to have influence on others and to let others have influence on you. To whom do you listen? Who listens (really listens) to you? Who do you make laugh? Who do you make mad? Who do you love? Who loves you?

_____

_____

_____

_____

_____

_____

_____

FREEDOM: Write down in this space the things about which you have choices. What choice did you make financially? What choice did you make about chores? What choice did you make about meals or clothing to wear or even which way to drive?

_____

_____

_____

_____

_____

_____

_____

_____

_____

_____

_____

_____

_____

_____

FUN: Write down moments when you had fun today. When did you laugh? What made you smile? What did you do that was creative?

_____

_____

_____

_____

_____

_____

_____

_____

_____

_____

_____

CHAPTER 6

A BRAIN THEORY, FOR THE MOMENT

Imagine for a moment you are sitting with friends in a very nice restaurant, studying the menu. Your waiter has explained the daily specials, all of which sound delicious and fattening. You are discussing with your friends the choices, relaxed and happy. All of sudden there is an explosion in the restaurant kitchen. Someone comes screaming out through the swinging doors yelling "Fire, Fire." Would you continue to calmly study the menu? Probably not. Instead, you'd probably make a mad dash for the door. Do you think you'll worry about what other people might think about you at that moment? Do you think you'd feel at all foolish? Probably not. You'll care about *surviving*. You'll worry about feeling foolish later, or never. That example illustrates a little of what this chapter is all about. Problem-solving by taking advantage of how your and your child's brain works.

THEORIES

You may or may not know there have been about a zillion theories about how brains and personalities work. People have tried to figure out other people based on their body types (for example, fat people are jolly), on the bumps on their skulls, on their astrological signs, or even on how well they process certain proteins. You probably have heard how people try to fit us into various categories like Type A or Type B, Lions or Otters, Passive and Aggressive, Phlegmatic or Sanguine, or whatever. There are about as many theories about how people work as there are people. I said all that to say this: I am about to give you a theory I learned at a conference I attended on the "Three Brain Theory". This theory is about as good as any you will read. And about as bad. And will likely be discounted within a year or so as new research shows up and "proves" it wrong (or maybe right).

Anyway, take all you read about how people and brains work with a grain of salt. Nothing is true for everyone and all research eventually leads us to new scientific "truths" that make our old "truths" almost comical. It was once believed by the very best scientific minds in the world that the sun revolves around the earth and that the earth is flat. It was once believed by the very best scientific minds that there are no such things as germs. It was once believed by the very best psychological minds that men's and women's brains are identical but that only our culture made us seem different. The good news about the particular theory I'll share with you is that it has been around for a long, long time and it seems to lead us to learning and problem-solving methods that really do work. My experience is that this theory is a very helpful way to understand how your child learns and how problem-solving might best occur in your home.

This book is about the difficult and angry child. Read this chapter carefully. You don't have to be a brain surgeon to understand the idea. It really makes common sense. However, keep in mind that it applies to everyone's behavior, to how they learn and how they problem solve – even you and me.

THE TRIUNE BRAIN THEORY, AS I UNDERSTAND IT

So, here's the theory: from a learning and problem solving viewpoint, our brains are built in three pieces: a Survival Brain, an Emotional Brain, and a Thinking Brain. Three brains in one, or the Triune Brain.

THINKING BRAIN
Challenge, problem solving, novelty

EMOTIONAL BRAIN
Feelings, relationships, having an affect on others

SURVIVAL BRAIN

Structure, Safety, Predictability, Rules

MY FAMILY'S BRAIN

The *Survival Brain* likes predictability, stability, safety, tradition, rules, structure and boundaries. This brain favors routine and wants things to be the way things were the last time. This is the brain that runs your morning routines. I like to get up early (a brief chapter on Early Risers is coming), have coffee, read, pray and exercise before my family gets up. I spent the first seven years of my life (before my brother was born) as an only child, so being alone is something I enjoy. If I sleep in, or over sleep, I'll still get up but my morning will feel "out of sorts" until I get to the next part of my usual routine (which is usually sitting in traffic on my way to work). I've also noticed that if I think I'm going to have time alone in the morning and my wife or daughter gets up early, too, I feel a little irritated until I get to the next part of my routine.

My wife, on the other hand, is the second of two girls in her family and she shared a room with her sister growing up. She doesn't like being alone. Now, as we all know, we always marry people different from us. Donna likes to sleep just as long as possible and then rush through the morning breathless. If she gets up early her morning doesn't feel right and she feels "out of sorts" until she gets to the next part of her routine. We have been married more than twenty-seven years and have had a running debate about the merits of getting up early and getting the day started versus the merits of sleeping in, getting lots of rest and starting the day later. Probably our Survival Brains will never let us really settle that debate.

Lindsey's brain, being that of an only child, is a lot like mine. Except she likes to sleep in, which I have never really figured out.

YOUR FAMILY'S BRAIN

You, too, have a Survival Brain. If you go to church, your pastor knows when you're missing because you're not sitting in "your" pew. If you always have oatmeal for breakfast and forgot to buy milk, you may find you can't think of anything else to eat for breakfast (in a kitchen full of food). If you are on vacation and it's time for lunch, odds are you'll pass up "Betty's Burgers," a local restaurant that may have the best burgers in four states, to go to McDonald's because your Survival Brain knows the food and atmosphere there are predictable. Traveling upsets your Survival Brain and it will only take so much adventure before it wants to get some routine back into life.

Your child, too, has a Survival Brain. He needs routine, traditions, predictability, safety and boundaries. More about that in the next chapter.

THE EMOTIONAL BRAIN

The next brain is the *Emotional Brain*. This brain likes feelings, relationships, having an effect on others and being affected by others. This is exactly what you think it is: the feeling part of life that drives our relationships. While the Survival Brain's impact is mostly unconscious, the Emotional Brain is both conscious and unconscious. Sometimes we know the emotional motivation for our behavior and sometimes we don't. It is fascinating to watch people who grew up in an alcoholic family go on to marry an alcoholic, even though they would tell you they would never want to do that. Part of it is the Survival Brain: it knows the alcoholic family routine, and part of it is the Emotional Brain – it has the skills to handle the feelings and relationships in an alcoholic family.

In my work with family violence, it's also fascinating to realize how many women who had been sexually abused as children grew up and fell in love with a batterer. There is something about the controlling man in both of those cases that was both predictable and appealing to some part of both the Survival and Emotional Brain.

It's also been fascinating to meet people who, according to what their childhood experiences taught their Survival and Emotional Brain, should have married alcoholics or batterers and didn't; or to meet people who did marry an alcoholic or batterer, left them and married someone who didn't drink or didn't abuse anyone. Nobody is stuck with their childhood brain. The wonderful news about brains is that you can learn new things until the day you die. The brain has the ability to build new learning paths if you develop new ways of thinking and acting – and practice them. *"The difference between where you are and where you want to be is what you do."* — Rev. Fulton Buntain, my pastor.

The Emotional Brain is considered the gateway to creativity. It fosters the kinds of creative thinking and creativity that results when different minds interact together. The old adage "Two heads are better than one" is really true. Teams of people who care for each other are often more effective at creative solutions than one person (The Marine Corps comes to mind). Corporations today often use team building exercises before they face difficult or complicated problems. You will do more fun things with your best friend than with a stranger, and most of your memories about the good old days probably include many relationship experiences that involved the Emotional Brain.

You will do better in life if you have someone close with whom you can share your experiences. I think that is part of why single parenting is so hard. There's no one easily available to discuss the tough issues. I also, always, recommend that parents make friends with other parents so you have someone to talk to about your child and yourself. Emotional support will make you a much better parent than you would otherwise be if you are isolated.

Your child, too, has an Emotional Brain that needs nurturing, support, and relationships. More about that in the next chapter, too.

THE THINKING BRAIN

Finally we have our Thinking Brain. This brain loves challenge, problem solving, novelty, stimulation and figuring things out. This is the brain that drives you to try new things, take a class, pick up a book to learn something new, have a new experience or even try a new hair style. This brain is stimulated by problems and likes to work on solutions. This is your (mostly) conscious brain. You and I tend to use this brain on purpose and can choose to consider the most complicated problems. This is where learning new skills and ideas takes place that, with practice, can become a part of our everyday routine.

When you travel to new areas or have new experiences, this brain is very happy while your Survival Brain is very unhappy. Travel with a friend or loved one and you'll find you'll often have a lot more fun than traveling alone because the Emotional Brain is now in the mix.

When we need to learn a new skill or need to solve a problem, we can't start the process if the Survival Brain is too uncomfortable with the situation because it will create an obstacle to learning. Consequently, we must begin learning or problem solving by starting with routines or structure to calm the Survival Brain. If things are not safe and predictable, we are not likely to learn or problem solve very well. I live in the Seattle area which is earthquake prone. Believe me, if I am out playing golf with good friends (using both my Thinking and Emotional Brains) and an earthquake hits (especially if it's the BIG ONE that's predicted), I won't care about my golf score or which club to use next. My Thinking Brain will quit. I also won't care which friend I leave behind on my way to some place of safety. My Emotional Brain will also quit. I will only care about my safety and how to survive the earthquake. My Survival Brain will be in high gear.

Under stress, when our Survival Brain feels threatened the first thing that seems to happen is that our Thinking Brain starts to shut down. We begin to make silly mistakes. We may begin four projects and not have one of them done at the end of the day. Our thoughts race, we toss and turn, we wake up tired. We may wake up at 2 a.m. thinking about things we should have been doing at 2 p.m. yesterday. I had breakfast with a friend of mine this morning. He is an engineer and his firm is doing very well. In fact, it is going so well he is experiencing a great deal of stress. He said he sat down yesterday and made a list of all the projects his firm is working on and came up with 29. He said the good news is he now knows what he has to do and can prioritize it. The bad news is he woke up at 3 a.m. this morning, couldn't get back to sleep and finally got up and just went to work on some things he'd brought home in his brief case. If you've ever overdrawn your checking account and tried to make sense of what happened you may have found you made the mistake on a particularly stressful day. You may also find, when you are under stress, the last thing you want to do is take on one more project or volunteer for one more job. The Thinking Brain is just done, finished, kaput. It doesn't want to think about new ideas or new jobs or new tasks. It doesn't want to solve a new problem or try a new hair style.

As our Thinking Brain begins shutting down, often our Emotional Brain seems to get busier. We get emotionally "messier." We get more emotional. We get more "touchy." We laugh easier, cry more, get angry quicker. We feel overloaded by relationships and feel people are too demanding. If the stress continues, we may make impulsive decisions. People report they will eat more, buy things they don't need (stay away from garage sales if you are under stress), even make disastrous emotional decisions such as having an affair. In our area a few years ago Boeing began to lay off a large number of its employees. Not long after the lay-offs began, banks started requiring Boeing employees to get a statement from Boeing that they weren't about to be laid off before the bank would grant a loan request. It was played up in the media as if the banks suddenly didn't trust perfectly trustworthy Boeing employees, but the banks were really just trying to avoid loaning money to people who, under stress, were using their Emotional Brains to make decisions. In this instance, Boeing would give an employee a "warn notice" which told him to expect to be laid off in 90 days. Occasionally an employee with a warn notice would run out and buy a new sports car or boat or something he or she could never pay for once they got laid off. The banks found they suddenly had a number of laid-off Boeing employees who had gotten loans just a few months earlier who now couldn't make the payments. The banks were experiencing the fall out of Emotional rather than Thinking Brain decision-making by people under a great deal of stress.

BACK TO THE BASICS

When the stress builds up to the point where the Emotional Brain itself is shut down we often find that people become depressed. They have something called a "flat affect" which simply means that they may appear unemotional. They don't want much interaction with others, they prefer to be alone, they may want to sleep a lot and they may have little appetite or report that nothing tastes good. They may move slower, seem to have very little energy and don't want to do anything that will require much work on their part. They are not much fun.

When both the Thinking Brain and the Emotional Brain are overwhelmed with stress, the Survival Brain seems to pretty well take over everything. People under overwhelming stress prefer routine and predictability. They don't want to be involved much in relationships and they don't want to try new and different things. You may have a friend or family member who has been through this and you want to tell them to "snap out of it" but you know that won't help. They just seem to want to get through the day with as little effort as possible. They don't want their routine interrupted or changed. If they are watching a favorite TV show, they may not even answer the telephone if you call in the middle of it. They feel swamped and you feel ignored. You both may feel helpless. A Survival Brain life isn't much fun and doesn't have much creativity. In a little bit I'll explain what you might do if you have a friend or loved one who seems caught in the Survival Brain lifestyle.

On the other hand, you've seen television news reports of some person who runs into a burning house and saves his child. The next time you see such a hero story, watch closely to how the hero describes his or her actions. It's always fascinating. Often the reporter will ask "Did you think of yourself as a hero?" Usually the answer is "No, I just wanted to save my child." Actually, if the reporter had asked the hero, "What were you *thinking* when you saw the house on fire?" The answer often would be, "Nothing, I didn't think about it." Of course not. If a hero thought about it, the Thinking Brain would say "Are you out of your mind? That house is on fire!!" So the Thinking Brain just shuts off. If the reporter asked the hero "What were you *feeling* when you saw the house on fire?" the hero would probably reply, "Nothing, I didn't stop to feel anything." Of course not. If the Emotional Brain got involved it would feel fear and prevent the hero from running into the house. So, it also shuts off. What's left is the Survival Brain which only cares about the safety of the child. When all else fails your Survival Brain will take over. That's why training for police and fire professionals is so important. They work under extreme stress and need to react "instinctively" to make the right decisions at the right moment. That's why you want an experienced pilot at the control of an airplane or an experienced parent to talk to when you are overwhelmed. They will have a different way of looking at a problem and finding a solution because they have "been there" before you and are more likely to be able to use their Thinking Brain to come up with a creative solution to the problem.

ANGER AND RAGE

Anger is in the Emotional Brain. It is just a feeling, like all the other feelings in your brain. The great thing about anger is that it can motivate us to use our Thinking Brain to solve a problem.

Rage, on the other hand (in some researchers' opinion) is in the Survival Brain. It is tied to survival, not to anger. We will often describe an angry person as being "enraged" or "in a rage" when he is, in fact, just very, very angry. A person in a rage will probably appear *unemotional*. Read the reports of a person who walks into his workplace and kills his supervisor. Usually he will be described as "cold blooded, quiet, machine like, mechanical" or such words. Rarely do you hear him described as "angry, yelling, swearing, out of control, red-faced" or with other such words to indicate anger.

Just after the terrible bombing in Oklahoma City had taken place, the first suspect was in jail. He was described as unemotional, silent, uncommunicative. He considered himself a prisoner of war and only gave his name, rank and serial number. People talked about him as angry or hating the government or some such descriptive phrase but, at the time of the bombing, I'll bet he was simply silent, focused, methodical and uncaring. I'd also imagine that as soon as he was arrested some police investigator was trying to befriend him, to touch his Emotional Brain, so that somehow, he could get to the Thinking Brain and find out the details of the bombing, about the other suspects, and about the important information so that the questions can be answered and other such incidents prevented. I sincerely hope that investigator was successful.

Don't believe your child is in a rage when he or she is just very angry. If he is red-faced and screaming, he is mad. If she is throwing a tantrum, she is mad. If he is spitting, hitting, biting, kicking or interacting with others, he is mad.

MAKE THE CONNECTION

In the first five chapters of this book we have looked at the kinds of stresses both you and your child can experience. We have focused on identifying and reducing stress so problem solving can be more successful. It is important for you to know when your child is merely angry versus when he or she is in a real rage. For small children, a tantrum may be a rage reaction, far more than just anger. He may feel his survival is threatened and will throw a tantrum that really is connected to his Survival Brain. For an older child, however, a tantrum is most likely a way to express anger and is only connected to her Emotional Brain. Handling our child who is in a rage is different than handling our child when he is merely angry, as you'll soon see. In both cases, however, you need to connect the stresses in your child's life to his or her attempt to solve the problem. If you can help your child reduce the stress he or she feels, the need to be angry – or even to be in a rage – will go away.

LEARNING, PROBLEM-SOLVING, STRESS AND THE THREE BRAINS

The theory is we learn in this order: first the Survival Brain, next the Emotional Brain, then, finally, the Thinking Brain. We "stress out" in this order: first the Thinking Brain, next the Emotional Brain, last the Survival Brain.

Notice a child who's lost in a store and you'll see the progression. First, she will try to solve the problem by looking around and calling for her parent, then she will begin to panic, cry, run or yell. Finally, she will begin to avoid everyone, she may suck her thumb and get very quiet. She began with the Thinking Brain trying to problem solve, then the Emotional Brain took over with more emotion, and finally the Survival Brain finished up with old, traditional behaviors.

You and I will also stress out in the same order. As a parent, we will find, as our stress increases, that our Thinking Brain will begin to shut down. Instead of being creative and thinking of a number of possible solutions to a problem, we seem to have a hard time concentrating and problem solving at all. Our Emotional Brain gets into the act and we find ourselves angry and upset. With enough stress we may find ourselves doing and saying things we learned as children, tapping into our old Survival Brain even though we never wanted to say or do those things to our children.

I have a friend, Chris, who is an elementary school teacher. She says she always wanted to be a teacher and grew up, went to school and became one. She tells this story: when she was in about the fourth grade she had a teacher who, as the class got more and more out of control, would begin to yell at the class and threaten them. She hated that and told herself "When I'm a teacher I'll *never* do that to my class." Her second day of teaching, as a student teacher, she found herself in front of her class, as it got more and more out of control, saying the very words she swore she would never say in the tone and volume of voice she swore she would never use. She had stressed out and gone back to very primitive, Survival Brain behavior. It can happen to any of us. The key is to not stop there.

In the next chapter I'll talk about discipline, which I view as teaching; and I'll be very specific about how to take advantage of the three brains in learning. However, before we move on to that, let me pull all of this together so it makes some sense.

MEMORIES

Remember back in Chapter One I said that an angry child is better off than one who is depressed and withdrawn? The angry, difficult child is usually that way because he or she is trying to *solve problems*, no matter how inappropriate their problem-solving behavior (hitting, screaming, etc.) may be. She is using her Emotional Brain, which is causing the feelings she is expressing. She is not far from being able to connect with her Thinking Brain.

On the other hand, the child who has given up trying to solve the problem may be apathetic, unresponsive, uncommunicative and even depressed, and is probably operating almost entirely from his Survival Brain. He is going to have a hard time connecting to his Thinking Brain and will not only have a hard time thinking of a good solution to the problem but probably won't care much whether the problem gets solved or not.

NOT JUST SHORT-TERM SULKING OR POUTING

If you believe your child is operating almost entirely out of his or her Survival Brain, it is critical that you get some outside professional help. Even very young children have been known to attempt suicide and you don't want to take any chances with a very depressed child.

GETTING BEYOND THE SURVIVAL BRAIN

The Emotional Brain provides the *motivation* to solve problems. That's why teachers are so crucial to the learning process. Good ones motivate us to learn while poor ones never seem to manage the connection. If you want to help your child get to his or her Thinking Brain, you'll most easily do that by going through the doorway of the Emotional Brain.

When your child is confronted with a problem to solve or a stressful situation that needs to be overcome, you need to help him by starting with the Survival Brain. You always want to start with the bottom layer of the brain and move up to the next two layers, in order. Sometimes, as a parent, you'll be able to change the situation and reduce the stress. Other times, however, your child will need to find a way to solve the problem or reduce the stress himself. One of the most difficult decisions facing a good parent is deciding which problems to solve for your child and which ones to let him handle on his own. He needs both experiences in order to grow up successfully. If you solve all of his problems for him, he'll never *learn* to solve his problems on his own. If you never help him solve his problems, he will face so many defeats he may never *believe* he can solve his own problems successfully. In the first case, the Thinking Brain is not allowed to really work and, in the second case, the Emotional Brain is never satisfied.

SIT BACK, RELAX, LET YOUR IMAGINATION WORK

Let me see if I can put all of this in context. We'll look at this more specifically in the next few chapters but it might be nice if we stepped back for a moment and looked at the whole picture rather than at only each of the parts.

Let's assume your child is facing some kind of stress at school and it's showing up as a behavior problem such as his unwillingness to get out of bed in the morning and get ready on time.

Going back to Chapter One, remember, put on the oxygen mask of self control first, before you try to deal with this behavior. Remember the importance of being *Internally* Controlled not *Externally* Controlled. The first step is always with ourselves, before with deal with our child. In this example, how do you define success as a parent? Is it having a child who is on time for school because that is an important value in your family or is it having a child who is on time for school because you don't want others (his teachers, your carpool, etc.) to think of you as a parent who lacks control of your child? When you answer that question, then you can answer this one: "What am I doing to be the parent I want to be in this situation?" That will help you stay Internally Controlled.

In Chapter Two we talked about memories and how feelings are remembered long after the facts have been forgotten. Look again at the list of feelings you made that you want your child to feel when he or she is dealing with you. In this example, what is the feeling you want your child to have about you to start the day? What feeling do you want to have about yourself to start the day?

In Chapter Three we talked about your stress and how important it is to have a good, daily Self Care program. In this example, ask yourself if *you* are under any undue stress and if you have been following a good Self Care routine. If you are under a lot of stress, take a moment to relax before you deal with your child. If you haven't been following a good Self Care routine, take a moment and be sure you have at least eaten something and have moved around (using your leg muscles to burn off some energy) before you deal with your child.

In Chapter Four we talked about your child's stresses and I asked you to make a list of the kinds of things your child might experience. Now is a good time to review that list to see if you can identify something specific that may be causing your child's behavior. Obviously, it also pays to have spent some time talking to your child to find out if he can help you identify the problem, too.

In Chapter Five we talked about the Four Basic Psychological Needs: Belonging, Power, Freedom, and Fun. Remember how important it is to meet the needs in sequence. On this particularly difficult morning, you would begin by reminding your child she Belongs to you. You and she are going to work on this problem, whatever it is, *together*. Once you have established that, you want to help her meet her Power needs. You need to let her influence you. You can do this by listening to her and telling her how badly *you* feel about the problem. It's fine to tell her you get angry and upset when she is late for school and how her lateness makes your day get off to a late start, too. However, your focus needs to be primarily on *her* feelings, not just your own.

The next need, Freedom, is the place where choices are given. It may be as simple as giving her this choice: "You can stay in bed until it is time to go to school and go in your pajamas or you can get up on time and go to school in your school clothes. Which would you like to do?" Keep in mind, with this need you must be willing to live with the choice. Offer only those choices with which you can live.

The final need, Fun, may not be met right then. It may be you will have to meet the Fun need at the end of the day. I do know parents who have made getting up and going to school a fun exercise by planning into each morning some activity their children enjoy. For example, I know one family who makes a game out of choosing breakfast cereal. They have three elementary school-aged children who, as a group, are allowed to make two cereal choices when they go grocery shopping. Each morning the first child in the kitchen, ready to go to school (which means clothes are on, hair is brushed or combed and the room is picked up with the bed made) gets to pick his or her cereal. That cereal can only be picked by one child. The next two children can only have the "second" cereal choice. This system has worked well for them, probably because they don't allow the first child up to "brag" about his or her victory. Eating the cereal is enough of a victory. I am wondering what they'll do as their children hit the teen years and looking good becomes more important than eating. Perhaps the first child up will get extra time in the bathroom, or something.

Now, here in Chapter Six I have added the three brain model. I've talked to you about moving up from one layer to the next: Survival Brain to Emotional Brain to Thinking Brain. In this example you would start by speaking to your child's Survival Brain. Be sure there is a routine that is predictable for your child. Did he go to bed at the usual time the night before? Did he get awakened this morning at the usual time? Did he eat breakfast? Did you touch him with a hug? If you have a "no" answer to any of those questions, you may have already discovered a part of the answer and you'll need to build those routines into the day. But let's say you answered all the questions with a "yes."

The first two of the Four Basic Needs, you'll notice, fit nicely into the Emotional Brain model about which I have been talking. Belonging and Power needs are what the Emotional Brain craves in order to move up to the problem solving part of the brain. Your ability to meet your child's first two Psychological Needs will dramatically improve his ability to solve the problem. In this example, meeting those two needs will help you and he define the problem from an *emotional* point of view before you try to solve the problem rationally using the Thinking Brain. The stronger the emotional bond between the two of you and the stronger your child feels about the problem, the more motivation you will both have to solve the problem. If either of you defines the problem, emotionally, as "no big deal," the harder it will be to find a solution to the problem.

A BRIEF ASIDE THAT FITS RIGHT IN HERE

Today, think about how much change has been brought about by small groups of people who worked together and had a strong sense of feeling about an issue. The emotional bond between them and their ability to make the majority of us have strong feelings about their particular issue has led to changes in government policies, as well as change in the way many of us live our lives today and in the very fabric of our society. The Sierra Club and Greenpeace come to mind, as do the patriots of the American Revolution and the people who started the *Make A Wish Foundation*.

NOW, BACK TO OUR REGULAR PROGRAM

The Thinking Brain comes to the problem solving process last. The Freedom Need that requires us to have choices is met by tapping the Thinking Brain. This will probably sound simplistic and obvious but there are only two solutions to any problem causing stress in our or our child's life. The first is to reduce or eliminate the stress itself. The second is to adjust to the stress that isn't going to change. *"You can't change the wind but you can adjust the sails"* (seen on a poster).

Your child can feel a sense of control just by looking at a problem from more than one perspective and developing a plan to either change it or live with it. There are some things your child cannot change. There are some things you and I cannot change. However, there is nothing you and I cannot adjust to, especially if we are working together with people who love us.

What do you do when you notice that your child is withdrawing or pulling away? Many times we will leave her alone and give her time "to get over it." We have a saying in our culture about how "time heals" and "absence makes the heart grow fonder." That idea makes good Thinking Brain sense but poor Survival or Emotional Brain sense.

For a person who seems to be moving into the Survival Brain mode of problem solving the best thing you can do is move closer to them emotionally. By increasing the amount of input into their Emotional Brain, you are more likely to access their Thinking Brain.

PUTTING THE PLAN TOGETHER

If your difficult and angry child seems to have gone primarily into his Survival brain to solve problems, you need to touch him Emotionally. It is important that you move closer to him, spend more time with him and talk more personally with him. You need to listen to him and feed back feelings to him. You need to let him know how his behavior affects how you feel. You want to combine the models I've given you: the Three Brains coupled with the Four Basic Psychological Needs.

If as a parent you are depressed and moving into your Survival Brain, you need to increase your time with others. You need to talk about your feelings. And you need to do something that affects others positively. You need to give yourself many opportunities to have your Emotional Brain touched.

THE BEST THINGS IN LIFE (AREN'T THINGS)

Life is richest if all Three Brains are honored every day. If you have routines, traditions and fundamental values and morals you practice every day, your life will be better. Added to that, if you have friends, family, pets, and give yourself to others to make their lives feel better, your life will be better. A friend of mine is a car dealer and he often tells his sales staff how important it is that the buyer has a good time. *"You never see a buyer sign the sales contract with a frown on his face."* – Jerry Korum. Finally, if you add challenge to your life, if you set out to learn something new, if you try a new experience every day, your life will be better. My grandfather died at the age of 93, a very happy, really wonderful old man. In fact, my goal is to live my life in such a way that I, too, at the end am a very happy, wonderful old man like him. He saw his oncoming death as a new adventure. What a way to go.

So, honor all Three Brains. In your relationships, be sure you are working to touch the Emotional Brains of your children and other loved ones because that's where you will have the most effect when you need it. Be sure, too, that your child and loved ones can touch your Emotional Brain because it is the gateway to creativity in your life. Above all, teach and model for your child how to live a balanced life where each of the Three Brains plays its unique role. If you are a successful role model and teacher your child will have a much better life.

SETTING UP THE THREE BRAINS FOR YOUR CHILD
EXERCISE — PART 1

Beginning with the Survival brain, write down the rules, routines and traditions for each of these areas:

WHAT ARE YOUR ROUTINES ABOUT?

Wake up time: _____

Bed time: _____

Play time: _____

Chore time: _____

Meal times: _____

    Breakfast: _____

    Lunch: _____

    Dinner: _____

    Snacks: _____

WHAT ARE YOUR TRADITIONS ABOUT?

    Family: _____

    Holidays: _____

    School: _____

    Faith: _____

WHAT ARE YOUR RULES ABOUT?

    How to treat others: _____

    How to treat animals: _____

    Lying: _____

    Stealing: _____

    Cheating: _____

    Respect: _____

    Homework: _____

SETTING UP THE THREE BRAINS FOR YOUR CHILD
EXERCISE — PART 2

For the Emotional Brain, what are the things you do to make your relationships work well?

LIST YOUR THREE FAVORITE SAYINGS OR IDEAS ABOUT LOVE:

- _____

- _____

- _____

LIST YOUR THREE FAVORITE SAYINGS OR IDEAS ABOUT FRIENDSHIP:

- _____

- _____

- _____

LIST YOUR THREE FAVORITE MEMORIES ABOUT YOUR BEST FRIEND:

- _____

- _____

- _____

LIST YOUR THREE FAVORITE MEMORIES ABOUT YOUR PARENTS:

- _____

- _____

- _____

LIST YOUR THREE FAVORITE MEMORIES ABOUT YOUR CHILD OR CHILDREN:

- _____

- _____

- _____

SETTING UP THE THREE BRAINS FOR YOUR CHILD
EXERCISE — PART 3

For the Thinking Brain, what are the things you do to keep learning, challenging yourself and trying new ideas?

LIST THREE THINGS YOU HAVE LEARNED IN THE PAST 6 MONTHS:

- _____
- _____
- _____

LIST THREE NEW ACTIVITIES YOU HAVE TRIED IN THE PAST YEAR:

- _____
- _____
- _____

LIST THREE BOOKS YOU HAVE READ IN THE PAST YEAR:

- _____
- _____
- _____

LIST YOUR THREE FAVORITE GAMES TO PLAY WITH YOUR CHILD OR CHILDREN:

- _____
- _____
- _____

LIST THE THREE MOST CREATIVE THINGS YOU HAVE DONE IN THE PAST YEAR:

- _____
- _____
- _____

CHAPTER 7

"I ASSUME YOU DON'T BELIEVE IN ... "

Often when I speak to a group a parent or teacher will come up to me and begin the conversation with, "I assume, from the way you spoke today, that you don't believe in _____ " and then they fill in the blank with words like "hitting or spanking" or perhaps "negative reinforcement" (which, by the way, is a complete misuse of the idea of punishment), or even sometimes "yelling or ever getting mad."

My answer is always, "Well, I can't exactly agree with that," which sends some people into fits as they try to convince me of the error of my ways and sends others back to their partners or family with an "I told you so" look on their face. So, as you read this chapter about discipline, keep in mind that *I* don't always agree with everything I say, either. Ultimately, *you* have to raise your children, not me or your neighbors or in-laws or their teachers or friends or anyone else. As I said earlier, you and your children, just as I and mine, are in this thing together. They have your thumbs (or eyes or chin or teeth or shared experiences of a lifetime). However, I do believe, if you follow the formula I'm going to suggest and if you apply your own style and personality to it, you will find discipline can be a generally pleasant experience for you and your child. Besides, if everything was rosy you probably wouldn't be reading this book anyway. Remember the quote: "Insanity is doing the same thing and expecting different results." Hopefully, this will be something new and you will get truly different results.

"WE MUST BECOME THE CHANGE WE WANT TO SEE IN THE WORLD."
— GANDHI

Discipline. Oh my, a difficult word and one that is loaded with meanings it probably never really should have had. If your parents were poor disciplinarians when you were growing up, the thought of discipline might bring up all kinds of bad feelings. If you have read books and listened to various experts you might believe discipline is a straightforward series of steps. We talk about disciplining a child and self-discipline and often the first means punishment and the second means following some financial budget or diet and exercise program. Usually there are a bunch of negative feelings and thoughts associated with discipline and many of us try to avoid it if we can.

My view of discipline is that we are trying to make disciples out of our children. A disciple is a person who follows, with their whole heart, a leader. They embody the same values, they look at life with the same perspective, they spend their time and energy learning as much as they can and they carry on the leader's visions and dreams as if they were their own. They are not puppy dogs following a master, mind you. Oh no, they have opinions and beliefs, too, and can question their leaders to explain more or to share why they do what they do and they will add their own personal flavor to the leader's vision and dreams. But they do follow and embrace many of the same values, ethics, morals and behaviors.

Trust me, even if you don't intend it, your child is your disciple. Just as you followed your parents, he will follow you. A friend of mine has a congenital hip problem and walks with a very distinct limp. Years ago, unknown to him, his son, all of about two years old, was following him to their church pew one morning limping along, just like his dad. His son has no hip problems (and grew into quite an athlete) but he was trying out his dad's way of walking, as your child and mine will try out our ways of doing nearly everything. If your leader was trustworthy and loving and had your best interests in his or her heart, you will probably follow closely. If your leader was untrustworthy, spiteful or used you for his or her own pleasure or gain, you are probably following at a far distance and may have spent a good deal of time in life trying to find a better leader or role model.

Discipline is about teaching your values, ethics and behaviors to your child, on purpose. It will happen by accident if you let it, but an active leader or teacher has a chance to correct the mistakes and wrong impressions of those who are following or learning.

A MODEL FORMULA FOR DISCIPLINE

Let's assume one of the values on your list is respecting others. What can you actively do to teach respect? What can you do if your child begins to show disrespect?

Here's a model I would suggest for teaching anything that is important to you and that is important for your child to learn.

THE FIRST RULE:
Always, invariably, put the oxygen mask on yourself
before you try to put it on your child.

A. NEVER DISCIPLINE IN ANGER. Using anger in discipline is like driving your car using only the accelerator. You'll go very fast but you'll probably lose control and cause a great deal of damage.

B. THE STEPS OF TEACHING

1. Plan to repeat the lesson at least six times. Research tells us that anything we learn one time, 16 days later we will remember 2% of it. Anything we learn six or more times, spaced over a period of time (spaced repetition) we will remember 62% of it fifteen years to life later. That's why, when I heard a three-year-old girl singing "Itsy Bitsy Spider" in a restaurant last week, I still knew the words and could sing right along. Repetition, repetition, repetition.

2. Go back to the Three Brain model I talked about in the last chapter. Remember, we begin teaching with the Survival Brain. First, we settle down and structure the environment. I'd suggest you have someplace in your home where the serious talk takes place. You may not want it to be the child's bedroom, which you want to be a place of rest and peace, nor should it be some place like the kitchen where you are likely to be interrupted. However, what ever place you choose, use it consistently and as often as you can. When we get into the "serious place," our Survival Brain settles down and says, "Okay I

know what goes on here. I've been here before." That will make problem solving much easier. I'd also suggest you find some phrase you always say when your child is in trouble. You may already consistently use a line so your child knows he is in trouble. If you just listen to yourself for a week, you'll probably hear yourself saying it more than once. If you ask your child, he can probably tell you what you always say when you are upset. One of my lines is: "Okay Lindsey, I've had enough!" She knows that means I am serious. The phrase has the same effect, it is part of the Survival Brain's traditions and makes the problem solving more predictable. I remember my dad's line: "Hey!" My mother's was a little longer, she used my full name and then I knew I was in trouble. "Gary Wayne Benton!!!" That was my mom's signal to my Survival Brain.

Remember, too, your child's chart from Chapter Four on Sources of Stress. If your child is tired or hungry, discipline will not be very effective. If he has eaten foods to which he is sensitive, he will not learn well. If you are tired or hungry, you won't be much of a teacher. Be wise. Children are smart. They don't always need to be dealt with the moment they have done something you want them to change. If you say your line to let them know you are upset and then tell them you'll deal with them later when you are both fed and more relaxed, they will still learn the lesson and they will appreciate the important modeling you have done.

3. Tell your child how her behavior affects you. Don't blame her or make her responsible for your feelings. That's not fair. You and I choose our feelings. However, be sure she knows that when she starts being disrespectful you feel hurt and sad. The Emotional Brain needs to know it has an effect on others. This is also the time to speak to the Belonging need. Be sure your child knows you are in this thing with her.

C. WHAT HAVE I GOTTEN MYSELF INTO?

I was doing a presentation to a group of parents and told this story: When Lindsey was about 12 we changed churches and she got involved with the youth meetings that happened on Friday evenings. She had only one real friend at the church and we, of course, wanted her to meet other kids her age and get to know more than this one good friend. One Friday Lindsey found out her friend wasn't going to the meeting that evening so she told her mother she wasn't going to go either. Now, my wife knew it was important for Lindsey to meet new friends and it wasn't as if she didn't know a number of kids who would be there. So Donna told Lindsey she was, too, going and Lindsey got mad. I, innocently on my way home from work, knew nothing of the war of the wills going on between the two powerful women in my house.

I drove into our driveway. We have an electric garage door opener. When I pushed the opener button and watched the door slowly rise, I could see, first, Lindsey's feet, then legs, then body, then tightly crossed arms and, finally, a very angry face. I thought "Oh-oh, what is going on now?"

As I walked into the garage, Lindsey began to tell me just how terrible and unfair her mother was for making her go to the youth night without her best friend. I listened, sent her to her room to settle down and went and looked up Donna, who explained what I already knew: it was time for Lindsey to go to the youth meeting on her own. Of course, I agreed. We had talked about her need to expand her friends a number of times.

So, I walked into Lindsey's room. All I managed to get out was, "I've talked to your mom ..." Lindsey blew up, "You're going to take her side, aren't you!?!"

(At that moment I remember thinking to myself, "Let's see, Lindsey, you are 12 and will be leaving me in about 6 or 7 years. I want to spend the rest of my life with Donna. You bet I'm going to take her side.")

So I said, "Well, yes."

That was it. Lindsey threw herself on her bed and said "I hate you, I hate you."

Now, I have to be honest. I began to giggle. It took us a long time to get pregnant and we only have the one child so I am thankful to be a dad. At that moment I thought to myself: "You get it all with children. The highest highs and the lowest lows. If I'd never been a dad I wouldn't have had this amazing experience."

I put my hand on her shoulder and told her how much I love her and how much I enjoy being her dad and that it was time for dinner. She didn't take my giggling all that well but, after dinner, on the way to the youth meeting, I told her how much I hated going to social events alone when I was her age (I still don't really like to go alone, now) and how I knew this was going to be a difficult night. I also told her I appreciated her willingness to go even though her best friend wasn't going to be there. We were okay and the night turned out much better than she thought it could have.

ANOTHER VIEW

I told this story to the parents' group and a woman in the front raised her hand and said, "I would never let my child say 'I hate you.' That shows too much disrespect." And, to be honest, I'd never thought of it that way and I sort of agree with her. Now, at the time it happened, I didn't interpret it as lack of respect. I just thought Lindsey was mad and hungry and trying to get a reaction out of me. And, since then, Lindsey has never said "I hate you" to either of us again. But, my feelings are not the same as yours or anyone else's. I interpreted "I hate you" at that time as no big deal and, in our family, it never became one. But other families are not like that. If you react to things your child does, be sure they are things important to you. I know parents who react to trivial things and seem to sort of ignore the really big ones. Make sure your values are visible to your children.

OKAY, BACK TO THE DISCIPLINE (TEACHING) PROCESS.

4. Once your child knows how his behavior affects you (your Emotional Brain), it's time for problem solving. Now you are going to be speaking to the Thinking Brain in your child. This is the hard part because it means that before you try to teach your child a better way of acting, you, too, will have to use your Thinking Brain.

Teaching is fairly straightforward. We introduce an idea, we explain the idea, we tell a story to illustrate the idea, we ask for feedback from the student about the idea and we reward the learning.

Learning is also fairly straightforward. We learn the idea, we practice the idea and we get rewarded for knowing or doing the idea.

Unlearning is equally straightforward. When we demonstrate a wrong idea, we are either not rewarded or we are punished or ignored for the wrong idea and we stop doing the wrong idea.

Child discipline is a matter of:

> 1. helping a child *unlearn* a wrong idea,
> 2. *teaching* a new idea to take its place and
> 3. *rewarding the learning.*

Now, I know that sounds far more academic than it seems to be in real life. However, what I've laid out is quite accurate. Let's see if I can illustrate it with a real life example.

OH HAPPY DAYS! A SPITTER!

Let's assume you don't want your child to spit on others because it is one of the worst forms of disrespect. Now, spitting is not unusual for young children and, while it causes others discomfort and parents embarrassment, it is not a fatal flaw.

Step one, of course, will be to put the oxygen mask on yourself, first. Take a breath, make sure you're ready to teach a new way for your child to solve whatever problem he is trying to solve by spitting.

Step two will be to help the child unlearn the spitting idea. Remember, there are three ways to help a child unlearn an idea: ignore it, don't reward it, punish it.

Ignoring a young child's behavior is a very powerful way to change it. Your child will try out a bunch of behaviors and will keep those that seem to work to help him meet his needs. I have a friend whose three year old girl learned a very bad word from people in their neighborhood. Of course, she came home and shared this new learning with her family, in front of guests from their church. My poor friends wanted to die. And, boy, did they react!

Well, their little girl, who, if there is justice in the world will have a child just like her of her own some day, found all that attention just a wonderful reward and began saying the bad word at every opportunity. They spanked her, they used time out, they told her how wrong it was, all to no effect. Finally they talked to a wise Christian counselor who told them the truth: the word was getting so much attention and making this little girl so powerful in the family, she wasn't likely to stop. His advice was to just ignore it and, lo and behold, it went away (but it took an uncomfortably long time).

Remember the four basic needs from Chapter 5: Belonging, Power, Freedom, Fun. If spitting gets no reaction from you or others, it moves down the list from power to probably fun and your child can replace one kind of fun with another and will move on from spitting to other things.

So, ignore what you can. Most good or bad behavior goes away if it is ignored long enough.

REINFORCEMENT, DEFINED

Let's say you can't ignore it. So, the next step is: don't reinforce it. Reinforcement is any reward that is likely to make the behavior happen again. Positive reinforcement means you *add* something to *increase* the likelihood of the behavior and negative reinforcement means you *take something away* to *increase* the likelihood of a behavior. A paycheck is a reward that is likely to make you and me go to work again. Shrimp curry on rice (which I dearly love) has a taste that is likely to make me eat it again. A kiss from my wife when I come home from work is likely to make me come home again. You get the picture. Those all add something I want or need to increase the likelihood of the behavior. Taking aspirin to reduce a headache, if it works, is an example of both positive and negative reinforcement. The aspirin's effect is to take away pain. If the headache goes away you are likely to take aspirin again. A reward is simply anything that improves the likelihood a behavior will happen again.

ONE SMART TEACHER

Obviously, ignoring a behavior is a way to not reward it. Another is to have an unexpected reaction to the behavior. A pre-school teacher shared this idea with me: when she has a spitter in her class she has an unexpected reaction. She *laughs* with delight and says "Oh, you like to spit. How wonderful. I love spitters." And then she marches her wonderful, newfound spitter into the bathroom and has him spit into the toilet until he can't spit any more. All the while encouraging him to continue spitting and letting him know he will get to do this every time he spits on anyone. She never has a spitter for more than a couple of days in her class.

One thing that we have found is unexpected reactions that include *humor* are far more effective than ones that don't. Don't give an unexpected reaction if you can't have some fun with it. My giggling when Lindsey said "I hate you" was an unexpected reaction with humor. And, whether you approve or disapprove of how I handled that situation (I'm not sure I approve of how I handled it either) it did get the effect I was hoping to get. Namely, the "I hate you" behavior stopped which was, of course, my goal. I heard an athlete talking on the radio about an "ugly win." He said he didn't care how they won so much as winning. In this case my reaction brought a win, even though others might define it as an "ugly win."

PUNISHMENT, DEFINED

Okay, so ignoring doesn't work; not rewarding doesn't work; and so now we get to punishment. Punishment is anything that *reduces* the likelihood the behavior will happen again. In the strictest definition, ignoring a behavior would be considered punishment. So would an unexpected reaction since both are likely to reduce the behavior.

If you go to a store and buy a product that turns out to be defective and the store refuses to refund your money, you are unlikely to shop in that store again. The store *punished* you. If you get pulled over by a policeman and he gives you a ticket for going too fast on a street, you are unlikely to speed on that road again, at least for awhile. The ticket was a *punishment*.

There are two ways to punish: add something or take something away. A traffic ticket is an example of adding something; losing money to a store is an example of taking something away.

With children, spanking is an example of adding something (pain) as a punishment; losing a toy or privilege is an example of taking something away.

POWERFUL REWARDS = POWERFUL PUNISHMENTS

The most powerful reward for people is *approval*. In fact you and I will work harder for approval than we will for money. We will give more time, more willingly and enjoy it more if we get approval than if we get paid. Believe that? Here's an example. I have a good friend who is a very successful engineer and a very good singer. He sings in our church choir and participates in our Christmas production every year. He will slow down his business for nearly a month and spend untold volunteer hours working on the Christmas production. He loves doing it, too, even though it is stressful. He is getting all four of his psychological needs met by being a part of the production team. He Belongs, he has Influence (Power), he is able to be Creative (Freedom) and he has Fun. He is being powerfully rewarded and gets approval all over the place.

Think about bosses you have had (or parents or teachers or coaches) who really appreciated what you did for them. Remember how much easier it was to go to work for them than for bosses who didn't seem to appreciate your work? Often it is difficult to leave such a boss and, if you are fortunate, perhaps you still keep in touch.

I have a friend who is a Marine. He hasn't been in the service for more than 25 years now, but he is still a Marine. He gave four important years of his life to the Marines and experienced high approval. He will go to his grave a Marine in his heart.

A smile, a thank you, a compliment, a hug are powerful forms of approval. Take advantage of every opportunity you have to give them away.

THE OTHER SIDE

Disapproval, therefore, is a powerful punishment. In truth, most forms of punishment are ways for one person to tell another they disapprove of their behavior. If you have more than one child you may have one who will change her behavior if all you do is frown at her. It takes a small amount of disapproval to provide motivation for change. On the other hand, you are reading this book because you have a firespitter and I'll bet you believe no amount of disapproval will ever change his behavior. So, you probably have gone to some extreme attempts to disapprove of his behavior. You may be hitting him, yelling at her, trying to find someone else to raise him, crying yourself to sleep at night over her or asking God (who created him just the way He wanted him) to change him.

THE MOST IMPORTANT IDEA IN THIS CHAPTER

Let me share a secret with you: **Disapproval is more effective when you give a lot of approval.** In fact, the more *approval* you give to your child, the more *effective* disapproval will become. A white sheet of paper looks much brighter on a black background than it does on a gray background. Disapproval stands out in stark **contrast** if your child has experienced mostly approval from you. The problem for many parents of firespitters is that they spend more time disapproving of their difficult child than approving, so the power of disapproval begins to fade.

SPANKING

As I mentioned, I have spent years working in the field of domestic and family violence. I have an opinion about spanking. My experience is that no matter what lesson you want to teach with spanking, two lessons are *always* taught whether you want to teach them or not:

 1. If you are in a position of power or authority, hitting is okay;
 2. When all else fails, hitting is acceptable, even hitting those you love.

Spouse abuse and child abuse both have their roots in the two lessons I have just listed. I have worked with hundreds of people who hit the people they love and both of those beliefs were in their minds when they abused others. Remember, we are trying to raise successful adults. Do you want your child to grow up believing either of those two beliefs? He or she will live out the value system which you believe and demonstrate.

THEN AGAIN...

That said, I also believe it is comforting for a child to believe his or her parent is powerful and able and willing to set physical limits. I am not suggesting you only talk to your firespitter in an attempt to change his or her behavior or to demonstrate your disapproval. That's ridiculous and not very effective. You've probably met parents who believe they can change a small child's behavior by simply reasoning with him. You've probably also correctly concluded that these are not very effective parents. Small children, especially, respond very much to touch, so touch needs to be a part of your discipline routine with them. The trick is to find effective, physical ways to limit a child's behavior without hitting him or her.

VARIETY IS THE SPICE OF LIFE (AND LEARNING)

In all areas of teaching, learning seems to take place sooner if the learner is taught in more than one way. With discipline, you'll find you are more successful if you teach in more than one way. For example telling *and* showing a child how to act is more helpful than just telling *or* just showing. With discipline, doing something physical *and* verbal will make the lesson easier to learn.

I would suggest, especially for young children, holding a child as you talk to him or her about a problem behavior, thus combining the two things you want: a physical touch coupled with the verbal lesson. The key is to hold your child until they accept you as the teacher, the person in authority. That can be difficult with a very strong-willed young child and you have to make a commitment to holding your child until the fact of your authority is established. It may take hours but you'll know when. Once that is accomplished then you can go on to the teaching part of the lesson. You may find that your child will cry when you hold him. That's very common. Don't worry, comfort him and let him know that learning who is in charge can be very hard (this is a great opportunity to tell another, "When I was your age" story). You have every right to comfort a crying child, even if you know it's because of the power struggle the two of you are in. However, it is crucial that *you win* the power struggle. Your child needs a powerful, protective parent who will make it clear just who is the boss. Holding a child until you know *he knows* you are the boss is important, especially early. Also, as with all things, you may need to repeat that experience more than once, a lot more than once.

DON'T BE THE BULLY YOUR CHILD LEARNS TO FEAR

The key is to using holding to *establish authority*, **not** to be cruel or mean or to prove who is tougher. Nothing stops learning faster than fear. If your child learns to fear you, he or she will learn to avoid you and, later in life, you both will pay a terrible price in suffering. Your discipline needs to be an *act of love and care*, not a way to prove you are the boss so you feel better. In fact, **any discipline that is done to make the *parent* feel better, isn't discipline at all**, it's just plain mean bullying and this is being done because the parent is in a position to do it, not to benefit the child. You and I know parents who discipline their children because these parents are upset with life and don't, at that moment at least, care whether the child learns a lesson or not. An angry parent never disciplines with the child's welfare as his top priority. If you (and I can tell you I have) have disciplined your child when you are angry, you know what I mean.

FOR EXAMPLE, MY DAD OF WHOM I BECAME A DISCIPLE

Let me give you an example. I grew up with my dad and mom. There were some difficult times but I had a chance to become a young man while my role model, my dad, was a part of my life every day. When I was five, my dad was Superman. He could pick up things I couldn't budge, he knew things I didn't understand, he had answers for every question I could think of, he had money, he could drive a car and I thought he knew it all and could do it all. If I had lost my dad at that age, I would have been left with the impression that "real men" knew everything, could fix everything, were always strong, were always right, were always in control. On top of that I would have had the "media man" as a role model. Generally in the entertainment media, the biggest, strongest, smartest, richest man with the car (and often a gun), wins.

As I got older (and so did my dad, I now realize) I had some interesting disciple experiences. My dad asked me to work on his car because he thought I knew more about cars than he did. I became about as strong as he. I learned some things he didn't know. He made mistakes and would say so. His career got bumpy and I realized he didn't control everything. He passed along wisdom ("Sometimes in a mud fight you have to throw mud") and encouraged me to think independently. He worried. He cried. He not only loved me, he liked me.

I have worked with hundreds of men who lost their dads before they were ten and they are stuck, to this day, with the image of that father who could do and control everything. They believe, in order to be a real man, that they must be in control of everything, must be able to answer everything, and that they can never appear weak or foolish or emotional. How sad. And what a difficult spot it puts them and their families in if ever something happens where they might appear weak, out of control or foolish. *Often they use anger to cover their fear* of appearing weak or a failure. That is not a lesson you want your child to learn. These people are not self-disciplined, not Internally Controlled. Rather they are the disciples of a myth of our culture and are *Externally Controlled.*

Back in Chapter One I talked about the difference between an Internally Controlled and an Externally Controlled person. A person who is Externally Controlled believes other people and circumstances are responsible for how his life is going and how he is feeling. He thinks it is the things outside of him that control him. And, because he allows it, they do. A person who is Internally Controlled believes he is responsible for how his life is going and how he is feeling. He has the Freedom to choose his reaction to any event in his life, even terrible ones. The Externally Controlled person, however, feeling frustrated and helpless, tends to lash out in anger and even violence to prove to himself that he is *not* helpless.

I have worked with hundreds of angry people who felt that they were the victims in situation after situation. They believed they were being controlled by their loved ones or people in authority. They spent hours and energy trying to change people and situations over which they had almost no real control yet spent little or no time trying to change themselves, over which they have almost total control. Life is too precious to be wasting moments we can never take back – angry words and actions just to prove who is boss.

"YOUR JOB, MR. PHELPS, SHOULD YOU CHOOSE TO DO IT..."
— Mission Impossible

Your job as a parent is to help your child learn *self* discipline and *self* control. People who are self disciplined and self controlled live with the idea that they can consciously choose how to feel and react to stresses in life. The Internally Controlled person doesn't have an easier life or feel less stress. Rather, he or she makes it his or her task to meet each situation and each moment with the idea that his or her own self, not the outside world, is responsible for what he or she thinks, feels and does. Self discipline means I have become a disciple (follower) of my own values and beliefs and I can choose how to react based on my Internal values, not based on the pressures and desires of the outside world. I have the personal Power and Freedom to choose the best course of life for me. The lessons of self discipline and self control are learned by your child spending time with a parent who is self disciplined and self controlled and by you, as a parent, helping your child take control of his life if he cannot do it himself.

WHAT IT'S REALLY ALL ABOUT, AFTER ALL

Discipline, in the end, is teaching our values and beliefs and rewarding them as they become manifested in our children. It is, as with any great task, a long process filled with small victories and defeats along the way. However, if you look at your favorite adults today they are probably children of parents who carefully taught the values of their lives. A self controlled, self disciplined adult is our goal.

UP IN THE AIR AGAIN

I read somewhere that an airliner is off course about 90% of the time. However the pilot continually adjusts the course and eventually lands it where it was destined to go. That is probably true about parenting. I feel off course about 90% of the time and seem to be continually adjusting the course as I go, and as the winds of change take place in my child's life. But, like an airliner, oh the places we will visit along the way and what adventures lie in store for us. The good news about discipline is: nobody does it right every time and parenting doesn't last forever. Someday your child will have children and you will be able to shake your head and chuckle at his struggles, just as others are no doubt shaking their heads at our struggles.

LEARNING EXERCISE

It is important to remember that you cannot teach a child to *not*. You (and I) cannot teach a child to not hit, not run, not spit, not say bad words, not get up early, not cry, not anything. We can only teach a child to *do*. For example, if you know how to ride a bicycle, there is nothing I (or anyone else) can ever do to teach you to not ride a bike. You'll know how to ride a bike forever. On the other hand, if I teach you to drive a car and you find that driving the car is a lot more convenient than riding a bike, pretty soon you'll quit riding the bike and just drive the car. With children it is the same idea. If you want a child to stop a behavior, *teach a better behavior to replace it* and reward the new behavior every chance you get.

List up to 5 behaviors you want your child to stop:

- _____
- _____
- _____
- _____
- _____

Now, behaviors to teach your child to do to replace the behaviors above:

- _____
- _____
- _____
- _____
- _____

APPROVAL AND DISAPPROVAL EXERCISE

Find five ways to approve of each of your children. Think about their bodies, their minds, their spirit, their friends, their responsibility, their chores, whatever. A simple way to give your child approval is to use a statement like this: "When you do _____ I feel _____ and you make my life better." (For example, "When you take care of the puppy I feel good and you make my life easier because I don't have to.") List all the things you can think to approve of in the space below:

* _____
* _____
* _____
* _____
* _____
* _____
* _____

Now, do the same for Disapproval. Think of ways to disapprove of behavior for each of your children. The simple rule for Disapproval is this: be sure to tell your child how the behavior affects you. "When you do _____ I feel _____ ." (For example, "When you don't take care of the puppy I feel sad and my life gets harder because I have to do more work.") In the space below, list all the ways you can think of to Disapprove:

* _____
* _____
* _____
* _____
* _____
* _____
* _____

CHAPTER 8

"YOU DESERVE A BREAK TODAY"

Every family seems to be blessed with at least one early riser. If you're the early riser in your family, you know what a gift you are to the rest of your family. You get up first, turn on the heat, maybe make the coffee, make enough noise and commotion in the house to assure the rest of the family another day has truly dawned and function as the alarm clock so that the late risers have some motivation to get up in the morning (probably to shut you up). You are probably accused of being just a little too cheery and energetic in the morning for anyone's good. I know how you feel. I am the early riser in my family. And, from my parents' description, I was always an early riser.

My wife and daughter are not early risers. In fact, they only rarely appreciate the unique and valuable gift that I, as the lone early riser in my house, am to them. But I get an experience they don't get and, until they read this chapter, I don't think they even know I get it.

THE WEE HOURS OF THE MORNING

When Lindsey was brand new and still eating every three hours, my wife and I had an agreement that whomever was up last with Lindsey got to stay in bed while the other parent went off to tend to Lindsey's needs. So, we would alternate the maintenance work all infants require. Donna nursed Lindsey so my responsibility was to get up when she cried, change her, bring her all fresh and clean to Donna and, when she was done eating, spend a little time with her as she fell back asleep. Honestly, some of my favorite Dad memories are of those times at 1:30 or 2:00 in the morning when the whole house was quiet and cool and Lindsey and I were just left with ourselves for a half hour or so. It was a special time for me to be with her with no distractions and all of my attention focused on her.

Well, as kids do, Lindsey grew up and slept through the night and that time of our life is past. But, now and then, I get to experience a little bit of it again.

Being the early riser, for years I have, at times, slipped into Lindsey's room to just sit there for a few moments as she sleeps. I am surrounded by the important things in her life (and the general hubbub of clothes and stuffed animals and pillows and school books that are now invariably on the floor) and by the impossible to explain sense of being a father and part of the endless miracle of life.

Honestly, I do the same with Donna, too, from time to time. Other times I will wander into our living room and just look at the way it's decorated and see Donna's hand in every detail. (Now and then Donna wanders into the garage which has my unmistakable hand all over it, but I don't think she feels the same sort of pleasure I feel). As I write this is it is the day before Thanksgiving and the family is coming to our house this year. Donna has already set the dining room table and the living room is decorated. Early this morning I just marveled at the every day artistry that is a part of my life.

Firespitters are tough. They challenge us at every turn and they are powerful, goal directed (or misdirected) people. But they, as we, are a "work in progress" and now and then you need to step back and just marvel at the work, so far. Here are some suggestions for stepping back for a moment, getting some perspective and enjoying the gift your little firespitter can be.

SUGGESTIONS

1. Do what I do, catch him or her asleep. Boy, a child looks so innocent then.

2. Take some time to get away alone with your child. Take a drive, go out to lunch at a favorite restaurant, ride your bikes together and *listen* as he talks.

3. Watch her in school or Sunday school (or, better yet, volunteer an hour or two in her class).

4. Watch him play with his friends. All those skills of compromise and cooperation you wish he would exercise around you seem to show up with his peers. The lessons do sink in, eventually.

5. Ask teachers, friends and grandparents to describe your child to you. To this day I am amazed at how differently Lindsey's teachers see her talent and abilities than I do.

6. Keep a weekly journal of your child's activities, experiences, victories and defeats. Over time it becomes a story of your child's life and you'll see the incredible changes that occur as brief moments here and there add up. Honestly, a ten minute investment each day in perspective makes an enormous difference in your ability to keep on the oxygen mask of self control.

7. If you have a camera, video tape your child from time to time. It is amazing to not only see their growth but to realize they gradually do gain more and more self control.

You need to maintain perspective. If you believe, as I do, that "children are a gift from God," now and then it pays to step back and admire the gift. Because, as Ralph Waldo Emerson put it, now and then "a child is a dimpled, curly-haired lunatic," too.

APPRECIATION LIST

On this sheet, list all of the things you really like about your child or children. If you like their sense of humor, write it down. If you like how their hair looks in the morning, write it down. If you like how much energy they have, write it down. The more you write, the better. When the list is pretty full, start to share those things with your child. He or she will love to hear you tell them the good things about them that you really appreciate.

_____

_____

_____

_____

_____

_____

_____

_____

_____

_____

_____

_____

_____

_____

_____

_____

_____

_____

_____

_____

_____

CHAPTER 9

WHERE DOES HE GET ALL THAT ANGER?

Do you ever wonder where your firespitter gets all of his or her anger? Well, this chapter will try to explain where anger comes from. In the next chapter I'll talk about ways to deal successfully with anger. First, however, it is important to know something about anger. To quote an old medical adage: "Diagnose first, *then* prescribe."

SOME DEFINITIONS

RAGE: a **survival response** to real or imagined threat (Survival brain)
ANGER: an emotional **feeling**, that's all, just a feeling (Emotional brain)
ASSERTIVENESS: **setting limits on behavior** in order to improve problem solving (Thinking brain)
ABUSE: anything done to **hurt or dominate** another

Now, if you think about those definitions there is room for interpretation in all of them. If you re-read *Abuse* and think about what that means, it is a very broad definition and can include much of what we regard as "normal" behavior. Is arguing over which television program to watch, abuse? Is placing your child on restriction, abuse? Is your child throwing a temper tantrum in a store in order to control you, abuse? It depends. The critical question is: *"What is the intention of the person?"* I have known people who have argued over television programs, who have placed their child on restriction and who have thrown temper tantrums and they all were abusive. The parents, in those cases, weren't trying to make disciples of their children or trying to help them learn self discipline or how to solve problems. Rather, they were trying to satisfy their own needs to feel powerful and to hurt or dominate their child. On the other hand, in the vast majority of cases, no, of course not, the behaviors we listed don't really constitute abuse by a parent or a child.

GOOD INTENTIONS

It is important, as a parent, to evaluate your *intention* when you are struggling with your difficult and angry child. If you *intend* to hurt or dominate your child, you are probably being abusive. If you *intend* to set reasonable limits, create consequences for behavior, establish reasonable authority so you have a chance to discipline and teach effectively, then you probably aren't being abusive. I know many parents are becoming more and more concerned about how professionals define abuse and there is considerable fear in our community about how Children's Protective Services can become involved in a family's life.

A WORD IN THEIR DEFENSE

If you could see the kinds of things a Children's Protective Services (CPS) caseworker sees on a daily or weekly basis, you would understand their hyper-vigilance about abuse to children. I have worked closely with CPS in the adoption agency because one of the programs found permanent, adoptive homes for abused and neglected children.

I can tell you about children who have been burned with cigarettes by their parents. I can tell you about an 8 week old baby girl who was nearly choked to death by her father. I can tell you about a 3 year old boy who had been sexually abused in ritualistic activities. I can tell you about children who spend most of their time cold, hungry and living in a car while their parents spend their lives in a bar. We only dealt with about 30 children a year in our program. One CPS worker may deal with hundreds in a single year, year after year.

I am not suggesting there is any reason to deny families the freedom to raise their children. I am suggesting there are some children who need to be protected from their families. If their neighbors, friends, extended family, school and church won't do it, the children must depend upon the government to do it.

So, enough said about that. I am not concerned that you are abusing your child. Anyone with the motivation to pick up a book like this is already someone who is using the Thinking brain to solve problems and examining his or her motives and intentions about raising children. And that's good news.

Please take everything I say with a grain of salt. You always have to apply information about parenting to your life, your child and your situation. However, there are some things we understand about how anger comes into play in a person's life and why difficult behaviors occur. I think you'll find much of this rings true and may help you gain a perspective on your own and your child's anger. Remember, we are operating on the principle that you have to help yourself (put on the oxygen mask) before you help your child. Understanding the anger-behavior connection will be valuable in more ways than one.

THE ANGER FLOW CHART

This is a "flow chart" about anger. Next I'll explain each element. Keep in mind, anger is a *feeling*. Most often we are concerned with the *behavior* an angry child shows and, as you will see, we may be putting our emphasis in the wrong place.

CHILDHOOD EXPERIENCES

☐

SELF ESTEEM (SELF IMAGE)

☐

EVENT

☐

SELF STATEMENTS

☐

FEELING

☐

ANGER

☐

BEHAVIOR

☐

REACTION

EXPLANATIONS OF THE ANGER FLOW CHART

Childhood (or Life) Experiences are those things all of us have experienced while growing up. This not only includes all we have learned and experienced but also our individual genetic make up which forms part of our life experience. As you know, if you have more than one child, we don't all start out the same. Our abilities, attitudes and temperament all vary. Some children are more active and some more passive. Some are good at sports and others good at talking. Some walk soon, others much later. But all of our experiences add up, and continue to add up as we live our lives. All of our experiences leave memories in our Emotional and Survival brain.

Self Esteem or Self Image is how we view ourselves. A definition of Self Esteem I heard that I like is: "Self Esteem comes from an accurate appraisal of your strengths and weaknesses." None of us are strong in everything. None of us are weak at everything. We are a combination of strengths and weaknesses. However, anger is most often found in those areas where we have poor Self Esteem or a poor Self Image.

THE MANY SIDES OF SELF ESTEEM

You and I do not have a good (or bad) Self Image. You and I don't have good (or bad) Self Esteem. We have many Self Images and many senses of Self Esteem. For example, my Self Esteem about myself as a carpenter is very poor. I am a terrible carpenter. If I had to make a living as a carpenter I would starve in about two weeks. I think I have a genetic flaw about carpentry. Everything I do turns out remarkably different from the plan. On the other hand, my Self Esteem about myself as a softball player is very good. I love softball. I have been known to practice alone, in the cold rain of February to get ready for softball in the summer. If I have a choice of building a planter box or playing softball, I would be wise to play softball. Even if my team loses, I will feel much better about myself at the end of the day than if I had tried to build a planter box. Now, this is not to say we shouldn't stretch or challenge ourselves or our children to try new things. However, we will tend to enjoy those things that "come naturally" more than those things we have to work hard to do.

Your Self Esteem varies from situation to situation. You may feel good about yourself as financial planner and poor about yourself as a pie-baker. You may feel you are the best driver on the road but the worst driver on the golf course. You may feel you are the best mother in the world but the worst public speaker. Your image of yourself will vary, based on your childhood and life experiences. And so will your child's. And so will his or her brothers' and sisters'. We are all different, which is the beauty of people, after all.

Event is anything at all. As you know, with a firespitter it's sometimes hard to figure out just why he or she is so upset. Sometimes it seems your angry and difficult child just wakes up angry. You'll probably hear about the Event sooner or later but we won't worry too much about that just now.

Self Statements are those things we tell ourselves about the Events in our lives. They come with a variety of titles like: old tapes, baggage, wounded child, internal self talk, and a bunch of others. Basically, however, they are those things we tell ourselves based on our Life (and particularly Childhood) Experiences. Often an old Self Statement will contain a "should, must, ought, always or never" in it. Such as "I should always be in control of myself." Or, "I'll never figure out how to balance my checkbook."

Here is a brief summary of *Stages of Moral Development* as defined by Lawrence Kohlberg.

Stages of Moral Development describes how your child makes moral decisions. Each stage develops as your child matures. In the first stage, which begins with the beginning of life, how a child decides what is right or wrong is based on how the child feels. If something feels good, it is good. If something feels bad, it is bad. For example, consider a child in the first stage of moral development. If he burns his hand on a hot stove, he's likely to say, "Bad stove." Now you and I know the stove is neither good nor bad. It's just a tool to use to cook. But, because of the pain, a child is likely to define the stove as bad. Kohlberg wasn't trying to describe morality. He was trying to describe (and I think he did a great job) the process of *explaining* how our moral sense develops.

Stage Two is the stage where parents experience the "terrible two's." In this stage, for the child, if something pleases him or her, it's good and right. If something displeases him or her, it's bad and wrong. In this stage, children cannot imagine someone else's viewpoint. Consequently, if a child in stage two wants candy in a store and you, as his parent refuse, you are likely to have a very angry, perhaps tantruming child on your hands. Even though you may explain how it's almost dinner time and how candy isn't good for him and how, if he's patient you'll get him candy he can have after he eats his dinner, he still will be angry because his need and his view of how you should act are not being met.

Stage Three is that stage, just after the terrible two's, when children believe pleasing others is the good and right thing to do. This is sort of a wonderful stage because your child is likely to be cooperative. However, this is also the stage where lying becomes obvious. In this stage, pleasing you is more important than telling the truth. For example, if you walk into your kitchen and find your four-year-old daughter has spilled milk on the floor and you ask her what happened, she may say, "I don't know." Or, she may make up a story, "The dog jumped on the table and knocked it over." Now, you probably will talk to her about lying and about how important it is to tell the truth. She will probably agree with you and tell you back exactly what you said. Fifteen minutes later you hear a crash in the living room and find a plant has been knocked over and your daughter standing there looking at it. "What happened?" you may ask.

"The dog knocked over the plant."

"But the dog is outside! What did I just say about lying?"

"I should always tell the truth."

"What happened?"

"I don't know, maybe the dog was inside for awhile."

Sometimes parents think they are raising a child who will become a criminal. However, the stage is normal and usually doesn't last too long.

There is a danger in this stage and that is for children around adults who will take advantage of them, especially sexually. The line will go something like: "Don't tell your mom, she will be very sad (or mad). You don't want to make her sad, do you?" In my experience, the average age for the onset of sexual abuse is about six. Right in the middle of this important developmental stage.

Because children in this stage of development are focused on pleasing others, they may keep the secret even though it would be better for them to tell.

Stage Four is the "Law and Order Orientation." This stage is most obvious when your children are between the ages of about 7 to 14 or so. Some children get there a little earlier and others stay there a little longer but, in general, this is the stage of *rules*. Things are good or bad based on the rules and values of the child's important family, peer and social groups. This is the stage when the "shoulds" in life show up. Odds are your firespitter isn't quite there yet, although he or she may be beginning to get the concept.

Stage Five is the stage where peer relationships become an important part of morality. This is the stage where what other people feel becomes very important. To some degree, this is the stage for most societies since common agreement about rules and values is an important way for societies and groups of friends to form. For parents of teenagers, however, this can be frustrating. "Everyone is wearing those expensive shoes." "Nobody has to go to bed as early as you make me go to bed."

To fit into society at large it is important for a teenager to explore the values of others. This is a hard time for teens and parents but a necessary step to the final, sixth stage.

The Sixth Stage of moral development usually occurs in early adulthood. In this stage what is good and right is based on our personal internal value system. We may go along with the crowd in most things but, in some things, we simply have to do what we know is the right thing for us and our family.

If you are concerned and confused as a parent, it is sometimes easier to follow the rules: "When I was growing up children had to be in bed by 7:30 every night.." Sometimes it is easier to follow the crowd: "Everyone is taking that new parenting class and doing exactly what the instructor says about raising children."

But, keep in mind what I said earlier: no one has written a book about your child or your family. It is your life and your child. Take everything with a grain of salt and ask yourself, "Does this piece of advice fit with my internal, personal value system?" If it does, use it. If it doesn't, don't be fooled because it has made sense for others and is the currently popular way to go.

Generally speaking, a child can *understand* up to two levels above their developmental stage but *cannot make moral decisions* beyond their developmental stage. So, for example, a child in Stage three, where, as I mentioned, lying behavior is very common as a way to please others, can *understand* a Stage four explanation such as: "The rule in our family is we never lie to each other," or even a Stage five explanation –such as: "I feel really hurt and the trust in our relationship is damaged when you lie to me" – will still be very likely to lie again if he or she feels lying will be more pleasing to you than telling the truth.

GAMES PEOPLE PLAY

One of the nice things about having a child is all the entertainment value available. When Lindsey was about ten and right in the middle of Stage Four of moral development, I tried the following experiment. Her favorite game is *Life* so, when I offered to play a game with her, she promptly got out the *Life* game and we set it up. Just before the game was about to begin I announced: "I've decided to change two rules." Lindsey replied: "No, you can't." To which I replied, "Oh sure. It's okay. I'm your Dad, I can change the rules if I want to." Well, she went ballistic, announced it was "not fair" (a classic line in this developmental stage) and proceeded to try to correct my errant ways. I kept insisting about the rule change until she started yelling, "Mom! MOM!" at which point (as I'm sure you can imagine) the experiment ended and we played the game straightforward, according to the rules she believed were true.

THE SHOULD GAME

Do you remember, back in the first chapter, I talked about how, under stress, we "regress" or go back to earlier problem solving behavior? If you find yourself starting to use the word "should" in statements about life, you are probably regressing back to the ages of about seven to fourteen. "Men should be strong, women should be able to cook, children should be seen and not heard, the government should do something about crime, the schools should teach the basics better, the police should be chasing criminals instead of giving me a parking ticket," and so on. The problem with the stages of Moral Development is, while we may grow up and leave them, they never leave us. You and I can make our moral decisions at any of the six levels. Under stress, all adults and children are likely to regress to an earlier stage.

Anytime you use the word "should" you might consider whether or not you are regressing back to about the age of 10 to make a decision, back to the old "Law and Order" stage of moral development. In my work with battering men and women the "shoulds" showed up over and over. We called it sex-role stereotyping but, basically, all that meant is the men, women and parents with whom we worked had very rigid ideas about the way men, women and children should think, act and feel. Anytime someone important in their life stepped outside of those expected roles there was likely to be emotional or physical violence to try to force them back into the way they "should" be acting. Decisions were often made by the emotional brain driven by anger, rather than by the Thinking brain, driven by logic.

Be wise and examine yourself when using the word "should" in your day to day problem solving. If you find it is easier to quote the rules than to think through a creative solution, you may be under too much stress to be an effective problem solver. You might be better advised to wait a little, put on the oxygen mask and approach the problem later. Certainly, if you hear yourself saying (as I have said): "You'll do it that way because I'm your father/mother (and therefore the rule maker) and I said so!," you can be very sure you are not really functioning at the level of an adult but as a really big and powerful ten year old. However, *rules are very important to your child.* I'm **not** suggesting you abandon them. We'll come back to this.

FEELINGS

Feelings are those emotional states we feel because of what we tell ourselves (Self Statements) about the events in our life. You'll notice it's not the Event that causes the Feeling. It is all of our Childhood Experiences and Self Esteem that combine to create the Self Statement triggered by a particular Event. It is the Self Statement that provides the basis for the Feeling.

For example, if your child gives you a hug or a kiss, you are likely to feel good. That's probably because you have a Self Statement that says something like: "I am a good Mom (or Dad) when I get a hug from my child." The hug, itself, doesn't cause the good feeling, the Self Statement about the hug causes the good feeling. If you were standing in line at the grocery store and a stranger walked up and hugged you, you might have a different feeling. Especially if the stranger was drunk.

It's not the hug. It's what you tell yourself about the hug that causes the feeling.

There was an interesting study I read about the difference between abusive parents and non-abusive parents. According to the study, when their child cried stress increased for non-abusive parents and, when their child smiled, stress decreased. For abusive parents, stress increased in *both* cases. The theory developed to explain this holds that for abusive parents *interaction* with their child, good or bad, is stressful. This means that, for this group of abusive parents, most of their Self Statements about their child led to bad feelings.

The feelings I'd encourage you to watch out for when you or your child is angry are: fear, hurt (physical or emotional), guilt, sadness, shame, embarrassment, loss of control. There are hundreds of feelings, of course, and many of them can lead to anger. The brief list, above, is just one I've found where the feelings seem to show up frequently when dealing with angry people.

ANGER

Anger is a feeling, too. A *secondary* feeling. It may be the first feeling you notice but it usually is *not* the first feeling you feel. In fact, if you pay attention to your own anger and look for a feeling "underneath" it, you'll probably find that you are feeling a number of things beside anger.

THE GOOD NEWS ABOUT ANGER

In itself, Anger is not a bad thing. It motivates us to change the things in life we don't like. As I said before, you reach your child's Thinking and problem solving brain *through* the Emotional brain, even if the Emotion is Anger. Truthfully, an angry child is not nearly the problem later in life as a child likely to be silent, unwilling to talk or solve problems. Angry children are attempting to solve a problem. Anytime your child is angry, be thankful. He or she is a problem *solver*, not a problem *maker*. His attempts may need some work and he can be frustrating to try to help, but he is motivated to change something in his life and that is good news. I believe America's patriarchs such as Nathan Hale and people of more recent history such as Dr. Martin Luther King and Mahatma Gandhi were all angry men. I know Helen Keller was an angry child. But, when we look at their lives, we see problem solvers, not problem makers. Their anger motivated them to change what they could, and the world changed because of them.

BEHAVIOR

Behavior is what your child does when he or she is angry. Often this is the first indication you have that your child is angry. You probably bought this book because of the way your child *acts* when he or she is angry. This is the <u>last step</u> in the flow chart that involves your child. The next step involves you. When I give you an example of a real life experience with this flow chart in a minute or so, I hope you'll come to realize how late in the process the behavior really is. At the end of the process, the *behavior* is what we see to let us know there is a problem that needs to be solved. However, don't be fooled into thinking that, because you don't see any uncomfortable behavior, there isn't a problem. Many times parents have successfully eliminated problem *behaviors* from their children only to raise very troubled adults. "He was a nice boy growing up, never any trouble," said a neighbor quoted in a news article about a serial killer.

YOUR CHOICE

I'll come back to this in the next chapter but I want you to think about this question for a minute or two. What are the *acceptable* ways for your child to express his or her anger? You can probably think of many unacceptable ways but you **must** have some acceptable ways. Remember what we said about discipline in chapter 7. Not only must you punish the behavior you don't want, you must also teach and reward the behavior you do want.

REACTION

Reaction is your part of this flow chart. You must react to how your child acts when he or she is angry or your child will not have any idea if he or she is doing it right or wrong. It is important to react in such a way that your child's Thinking Brain is reached. In all anger management programs, the Reaction step is the first step to treatment. The stronger the reaction, the more likely treatment will be successful. Studies show, for adults who commit crimes, the very best Reaction is going to jail (even if only for a day). The Reaction provides motivation for the person to change his or her behavior.

With children, your Reaction is very important. Be sure to get upset about things that are really upsetting. Remember how important *contrast* is in discipline. If you over-react to everything, your child won't know for sure what is really important and what is not. When that happens your Reaction will not have the effect of helping your child learn better ways to handle anger and solve problems.

I mean this: *You are your child's best hope for success in life.* React accordingly.

For Example:

I'm going to give you a personal example about me as an adult and, in the next chapter, an example of a four year old child. Since we always start with ourselves first, I'm starting with me.

If you met me you would notice I am not a large person. In fact, growing up, there were two Garys in my grade school, Gary Mitchell and me. In order to distinguish us, our friends called him "Gary" and called me "little Gary." How cute.

Anyway, being a boy, growing up in the fifties, there were grade school fights (not much has changed in 40 years, except we didn't carry weapons). Now, being small I learned to be a student of fights because I needed to figure out how to survive one if I ever got into it. This is what I learned as a boy: grade school fights have certain steps:

Step 1 is name calling and threatening,
Step 2 is pushing and shoving,
Step 3 is wrestling, and
Step 4 is punching.

I learned, quickly, if the fight got much beyond name calling and threatening, I would lose.

I had two valuable skills growing up. First, I was a very fast runner. Second, I made friends with big kids. So, in order to survive grade school fights, I cut out the middle steps. If someone called me a name or threatened me, I didn't play the game. I didn't threaten back, I didn't call names, I didn't push and shove or wrestle. Instead I went immediately to step 4 and punched him, and ran fast, toward my big friends. Now, I wasn't very big and I didn't do much damage but it worked. I learned, in my *Childhood Experiences*, to over-react aggressively. That was a very useful skill in grade school. I got a reputation for being just a little off-kilter and so avoided many fights because I was just too unpredictable.

My *Self Esteem* was good about myself as a runner and cultivator of big friends, but poor about myself as a fighter.

We'll ignore the *Event* for a moment.

My *Self Statement* is,"I should never be threatened" (from my Survival Brain.)

My *Feelings*, when my Self Statement doesn't line up with reality are: fear, threatened, out of control.

My *Anger* is real and a motivator to do something about the problem, as I see it.

My *Behavior* is to over-react aggressively.

The *Reaction* is hard to predict, it will vary by the situation of which I am a part.

HERE'S AN ABSOLUTELY TRUE STORY

(the names have been changed, of course)

I was a family therapist working for a very nice non-profit, family counseling agency in one of their suburban branch offices. I'd finished my Master's degree and had been there about a year. I had spent six years prior to that position working in a group home with pre-delinquent, emotionally disturbed teen age boys.

One Friday afternoon, just as I was locking up the office to go home, the telephone rang. I, being the first born and overly responsible one in my family, answered it. A 15 year old boy, Bill, was on the other end of the phone and he proceeded to tell me he was going to run away from home.

Bill had gotten our agency's phone number out of the Yellow Pages under "Family Counseling." He lived about an hour and a half away, by bus, in another suburban neighborhood. He was only about a half hour away by car.

I had worked with a lot of 15 year old boys in my professional life to that point and I knew running away is a dangerous idea. I'd known many boys who had been abused and hurt on the streets. My first goal was to talk him out of running away and the second, if that failed, was to send him to someplace safe until someone could work with his family.

He began to tell me about his family and as he began to describe them I realized I knew him. He was the step-son of a man on my softball team the previous summer. Actually, I sort of agreed with him. I, too, thought he had pretty poor parents based on my experiences with his step-dad and mother.

Anyway, as we continued to talk he realized he knew me, too. All of a sudden he just stopped the conversation and said:

"Hey, I think I know you."

I replied, "I think you do."

"You know my Dad!!"

"Yes, I do."

"If you tell my Dad I called you, so help me, I'm going to come down there and kick your —-. I know karate, I know judo. You're just a punk, shrimpy little guy ..." and on he went.

Boy, I'll tell you I was **MAD**. My knuckles turned white on the phone handset, I gripped it so hard.

I yelled: "If you think you're so tough, come on down," and I slammed the phone back on the receiver.

Now, that was a very professional response, don't you think? A full grown therapist telling a 15 year old to "come on down." The boy would have to get on a bus, travel 45 minutes to Seattle, transfer buses, travel back to my community another 45 minutes, and I was on my way home anyway. Good grief.

What happened to me is very simple. I traveled the Anger Flow Chart. My stress was high (it was the end of the day at the end of a very long week). I was tired. I was hungry, and I didn't put on the oxygen mask. The threat tagged the old Self Statement I had developed in grade school, based on my Childhood Experiences and Self Image. The Self Statement generated Feelings, which generated Anger, which generated truly stupid Behavior, the Response to which left me feeling lousy and guilty all weekend.

By the way, the story does have a happy ending. He didn't run away after all. He stayed home, talked to his school counselor on Monday and he and his family began seeing a counselor in their area. No thanks to me.

GETTING OFF THE ANGER FLOW CHART

You and I and our children can travel the Anger Flow Chart in the blink of an eye. Nothing goes on in your body that didn't start in your mind. I didn't *react* to the actual threat from this 15 year old. Rather, I pulled out of my memory my old grade school experiences and reacted to those as I had trained myself to do for years and years. Although it was a dumb idea, it was still an idea that began in my head, not in the immediate situation.

One of the most important things research has showed about anger is this: While anger is a *feeling*, how we *express* anger is *learned*, largely by modeling or trial and error. Anything learned can be unlearned (or at least replaced with a better idea), so an angry child (or adult) can be taught better ways to use all that energy that's wrapped up in anger.

When you are angry with your child, look first at the Feelings you feel *underneath* the Anger. If you can change those, your anger will go away. If you want to do some self -examination, try to figure out what "should" is in your Self Statement. If you can change that, not only will your Anger go away, it probably won't really come up again, as least not in a way that feels out of control. If you want to do therapy on yourself, figure out what in your Life Experiences caused you to develop your Self Statements. Any time you feel angry, your best, first move is to examine yourself before you examine the Event you think caused your anger. You will be using your Thinking Brain to get control over your Emotional and Survival Brains.

ONE LAST STORY

As you can imagine from my example, I am not very good at being threatened. My response to threat is to be aggressive. My Self Statements include at least one that says: "I should never be threatened." Let me tell you how that changed for me.

I was leading one of the anger management groups in my program. I was in a room with 10 men, all of whom had been court ordered for assault. We were talking about the things in life that triggered our anger and I shared that being cut off by another driver on the freeway really burned me up. A guy in the group said, "You're kidding. That never bothers me at all." Well, I thought, here's a guy who is certifiably angry and he doesn't get as upset as I, the therapist, do in traffic. So I asked, "Why not?" "Well," he replied, "I have a loaded gun under the seat in my car. If someone cuts me off on the freeway I just pull up along side them, show them my gun and they back right off."

That did it for me. I thought to myself: "Angry guys are on the freeways and they carry guns." I dramatically changed my Self Statement that night and now drive the freeway feeling significantly calmer and considerably more rational. I don't feel threatened when someone cuts me off because, instead of saying, "I should never be threatened," I say to myself: "Is this stretch of freeway worth getting shot over?"

You can change your Self Statements about your child, your parenting and just about anything else that you decide is not helping you live your life the way you know is best. When you do, your feelings will change and, of course, so will your anger.

HOMEWORK

Carry around a 3X5 card (or two) and, *every time you are angry*, write on it what feeling you feel. This is a great exercise and will reveal far more than you might imagine. As well, in the long run it will really help you help your child.

DIFFICULT BEHAVIOR WORKSHEET

List the feelings your difficult child might be feeling when he or she is angry or acting up. Sometimes it helps to go through a dictionary or thesaurus to find feeling words. Keep in mind that we often see children who are difficult when they are hurt, afraid, agitated, shy, guilty, sad, embarrassed, stubborn, tired, hungry, overwhelmed, proud or even just really excited.

_____

_____

_____

_____

_____

_____

Now list the behaviors *you* might use to demonstrate the feelings listed above. Pay attention to how you hold your body, if you sigh out loud, if you cry, if you storm around, if you become silent.

_____

_____

_____

_____

_____

_____

Now list the behaviors your child might use to demonstrate those feelings. Remember, children are more likely to *act* how they feel than tell you using words.

_____

_____

_____

_____

_____

_____

CHAPTER 10

NOW WHAT?
HELPING AN ANGRY CHILD

All right. Now you have an idea of anger. It is not the Event that causes Anger but what we tell ourselves about the Event (our Self Statements) that cause the Feelings that cause the Anger. As you read this chapter, keep that in mind.

When dealing with your difficult and angry child, it is important you travel "up" the Anger Escalator. In other words, you start at the Reaction end of it and travel back to Action and then to Anger and then to Feelings and, maybe, even to Self Statements. This is where you, as a parent, get to put this all together.

STEP ONE

First, as I mentioned in the last chapter, write down three acceptable ways to demonstrate anger in your family:

1. _____
2. _____
3. _____

These will be the most important behaviors you will teach your child about being angry. Remember, *feeling* angry is a normal human experience. *Acting* angry is learned. If your child is going to be a faithful disciple, you need to teach him or her how to be angry in ways that will not cause trouble in your family.

For example, in some families yelling is perfectly okay. In others, storming off to a room is okay. For others, sitting in silence is okay. For others doing some kind of activity such as walking or riding a bike is okay.

It pays to take a hard look at how your family already handles anger. In some families, having a drink or two or more is how anger is handled. In others, name calling or bad mouthing others is how anger is handled. In other families punching a wall or kicking a door or furniture is how anger is handled. In too many families, hitting each other is how anger is handled.

You already have a way to let others know you are angry. If you find those ways are helpful and make for better relationships, teach them to your child. If you find some of those ways aren't helpful and your relationships are worse, you need to decide what is a better way to express anger and, not only teach it to your child, but practice it yourself.

A WARNING

I will tell you, based on my experience, any way you express anger that causes *fear* in someone else is bound to cause more trouble than it cures. People who are afraid make very poor problem solvers. Remember the Triune Brain model in chapter 6? The Survival brain needs to feel safe. If your child or others in your family don't feel safe around you, you will never develop good relationships and problem solving will always be difficult.

Here are some things that cause fear in most people, especially children:

1. *Unexpected noise (yelling, screaming or wailing, for example)*
2. *Being called names or being threatened*
3. *Hitting an object such as a wall, door or furniture*
4. *Being abandoned (a parent storming off in the car, for example)*
5. *Being hit*
6. *Watching a parent or sibling get hit*

Think of your own experiences growing up and the things that frightened you. Your list will be better than mine, I'm sure.

VALUES

The Reaction part of the Anger Escalator is where you get to teach your values to your child. What you really believe is the right way to live will show up in the very first step you take to help your firespitter learn how to be angry.

Where Did He Learn To Do THAT!?!

For example, if you believe in peace at all costs and you give in easily when your child (or others) are angry, you will teach the value of being a victim. Your child will grow up and very likely either choose to be a victim of other peoples' anger as he or she has learned from you or will choose to never be a victim, never learn to compromise and always react with aggression when others are angry. One of the most difficult things I find for many of my counseling clients to admit is that we only have one of two choices when it comes to problem solving: to do it the way we think our parents did it or to do the opposite. I can't tell you how many times I have heard a client say "I refuse to be like my mother (or father)," only to find, on examination, that they were almost identical to their mother or father. On the other hand, I have also had clients who were exactly the opposite of how they described their mother or father, but found their way of solving problems was no more successful. None of us know the middle ground in personal decision making, which is why we seek other opinions. Often we will look for someone who knows the middle ground when we are at one extreme or the other. If you don't want your child to act in ways you don't particularly like about yourself, you need to find a new way for yourself, first; then teach and model it for your child. Don't believe, for a moment, you can tell your child to act differently than you act. The old adage, "actions speak louder than words" – it's true.

So, know your values, talk about your values, live your values. If your child acts angry in a way that is inconsistent with your values, you need to follow the discipline model we talked about in Chapter 7. Remember, punish the behavior you don't want and teach and reward the behavior you do want.

Here are some things I would encourage you to always react negatively to:

1. *Hitting.* If your child learns it is okay to hit when he is angry, he will have trouble his whole life. Hitting brings an immediate response but causes long-term problems in every relationship. It seems to be the easy way out of a difficult situation but, in the long run, causes fear to be a part of every decision.

2. *Name calling.* If your child learns it is okay to call people names when she is angry, she will simply learn to dehumanize others with whom she is mad. It is sometimes called "objectifying" others. That simply means we stop thinking of people as people and make objects out of them. Objectifying others is behind every form of violence and discrimination. When we objectify someone we can then justify limiting their freedom, limiting their opportunities, and even doing them harm. Watch how terrorists treat their captives. They never let them be human. They are objects from the beginning. They never make eye contact, they don't find out about their families or hopes or dreams. Their victims are treated like animals, often not even allowed to speak. Racism is another example of making objects of others based on their skin color or national origin. It goes on everywhere, not just in America. I have a friend from a rural part of Viet Nam and he and his people were discriminated against because they were not of the same class as the people in power in his country. If your child is allowed to call people names she will learn it is easier to ignore other peoples' feelings and minimize their needs.

3. *Disrespecting you.* It is important your child has a parent who is more than a friend. You are the person who represents the values you want your child to learn. If he learns it is okay to disrespect you, he will also learn to disrespect your values. I've often talked to parents of children only four or five years old who were afraid to insist that their children follow their rules. When I asked what happened when the parent asked for some particular behavior (go to bed, pick up your toys, don't hit your sister, don't draw on the walls, etc.), I often found parents would give up trying to enforce the expected behavior. Instead, the child would throw a tantrum or refuse and the parent, after some whining and threatening, would give up. When you give up on the things that are important to you, you are also giving up on the lesson you want your child to learn. *There is little in life more frightening for a child than to find he is more powerful than his parent.*

THE SUCCESS FORMULA

Now, it is ridiculous to think one formula exists for successfully dealing with an angry child but I'm going to teach you one, anyway. Let's assume your child consistently throws tantrums when you ask her to do anything she doesn't want to do. For the sake of the example, let's say it is time for her to pick up her toys and go to bed.

First, keep in mind that your child is trying to solve a problem. Most likely she is trying to convince you to change your ways and not insist that she stop playing and go to bed. You, too, are trying to solve a problem. Most likely you believe children need a certain amount of sleep (not to mention you need a break) and that a predictable bed time is good for children. Your *values* are being challenged. The values about consistent living, about responsibility for cleaning up after oneself, about obeying authority. All kinds of wonderful lessons are available in this experience.

You also remember lessons taught with positive reinforcement are learned about ten times quicker than lessons taught by punishment.

So, you walk into her room and say "Jill, it's time for bed."

She promptly starts to whine, complain and pretend you're not there.

You start to insist. She starts to bargain, "Just a few more minutes."

You really insist. She throws a tantrum (not to mention the toy in her hand at the moment). She also throws herself on the floor and clearly defies you.

A little part of you wants to give up about then. Another little part of you wants to really show her who is the boss. A big part of you recognizes a strong-willed, tired little girl who should have been in bed a half hour ago.

Your only goal is to solve the problem of picking up the toys and going to bed. You don't need to solve the authority problem (that will solve itself).

First, speak to the *Survival* brain. Put your hands on her and move her to a restricted area of the room such as onto the bed, into a corner or firmly on your lap.

Don't say a word. Authority doesn't need explanations. When a police officer pulls you over, he or she doesn't need to explain who the authority is. It is clear to everyone because it is clear to the police officer. You are the authority figure, you don't have to tell anyone or prove it to a four year old.

When she has calmed down some, speak to the Emotional brain. "I feel upset when you throw a tantrum and refuse to pick up your toys and go to bed." Expect, now, another tantrum. You and she have connected emotionally and she will likely use this as an opportunity to try to get you to shape up. Stay with the Survival brain. Don't let go of her, keep things restricted and predictable.

When she has calmed down, again, ask her how she feels. Expect a tantrum, again. Hang in there. She may not be able to tell you any words at all so expect her to use some behavior to try to tell you how she feels. Anything she does to try to express her feelings is good news because she is trying to connect to your Emotional brain, too. The more feeling words you can teach a child, the better he or she will be as problem solvers when older.

All this time you are teaching important values. First, you are teaching who is the power and authority in the family (you if you don't give in). Second, you are teaching her that, even though she is angry and upset, you don't have to be. You are teaching the value of self control. Third, you are teaching her that you and she are in this together (she Belongs to you) and you will solve this together, sooner or later. Fourth you are teaching her the value of patience. Not everything has to be settled immediately. In fact, the more important the lesson the more time it often takes to teach.

Now, move to the Thinking brain. Remember, disapprove of the behavior you don't want but *always* teach and reward the behavior you do want.

There are three behaviors to choose to change in this little example. There is the tantrum behavior, the picking up the toys behavior, and the going to bed behavior. Decide which *one* is the most important and concentrate your energy on that *one* lesson.

Some parents are okay with tantrums as long as the work gets done. Some parents really want a neat and tidy room, even if it means the child goes to bed later than she was told. Some parents want kids in bed when they need to be in bed and don't much care if the room is picked up first or not. Some parents believe the tantrum is the most important behavior to change. Whatever is important to you is the lesson you want to teach. If all three lessons are important to you, pick the most important one first and then teach the others later.

I'll decide, for this example, that the tantrum behavior is the one I most want to see changed.

I will continue to hold my daughter and speak softly. I don't need to be upset with all of this, I need to solve a problem.

So, in speaking to the Thinking brain I'm going to say something like this: "I really don't like it when you throw a tantrum when I ask you to do things you don't want to do. If you throw a tantrum again you'll have to sit in the corner for 4 minutes." I have now given the disapproval for the behavior I don't like. If I get a tantrum, I'll put her in the corner for 4 minutes.

Next, since we are in this thing together, I'd say something like this: "When I was your age I hated to stop playing and to go to bed, too. I'll show you what I learned about how to handle that. This will be fun."

At that point, since we are in this together, I'd take my daughter and practice the behavior I want.

I'd walk out of the room with her and then turn around and come back. I'd tell her what I want her to do. "I'm going to come in here and tell you it's time for bed and I want you to pick up your toys. Ready?"

Now, if you want to be very wise and you have a very stubborn child, try this technique: tell your child you *want* her to throw a tantrum. It's an interesting problem for a strong willed child. If she throws the tantrum as you've told her to, you win because she is doing what you told her to do. If she doesn't, you also win because you don't have to deal with the tantrum.

Let's assume she throws the tantrum. Be happy, pick her up and give her a hug, thank her for doing what you asked, tell her you'll ask her to throw more tantrums in the future, just for the fun of it. Expect the tantrum to be very short-lived.

Next, teach her how you want her to handle your instructions to pick up the toys and go to bed. I might say something like this: "When I was your age and hated to stop playing and go to bed what I did was ask my dad to help me pick up the toys. Sometimes he did and sometimes he didn't."

Next I'd tell her to ask me for some help. When she did, I would say "No, I can't right now." Then I'd tell her to ask me again. When she did, I would say "Sure, I'm happy to help." All that's going on is teaching. I'm teaching it is okay to ask for help and it's okay for me to say yes or no. Right now all I care about is that we are so caught up in the lesson we have forgotten the tantrum.

By now we'd all be so tired we'd probably all want to go to bed. What I would tell my daughter is: "Tomorrow night I'm going to tell you to pick up your toys and go to bed. If you throw a tantrum, you'll have to sit in the corner for 4 minutes and then pick up your toys and go to bed. If you ask me for help without throwing a tantrum I might be able to help you and I will read you a story."

The trouble with learning is it usually takes six lessons before we really get the message. This particular lesson will probably be repeated six or more times before it sinks in. With an angry and difficult child, you have to make a commitment to teaching the lessons more than once. It can be frustrating and tiring and you'll often feel like you're running into a brick wall, but the values you teach do, eventually, sink in. You are raising an *adult*, after all, so the lessons you teach need to last a lifetime.

UP THE ANGER ESCALATOR

Using the tantrum example as a backdrop, we have simply traveled from the Reaction step of the Anger Escalator to the Self Statement step.

The *Reaction* part was really in two places. First, you decided how it is okay to be angry in your family. Second, you didn't get angry just because your child was angry. You stayed calm and reacted as you *chose* to react. You put on the oxygen mask of self control before you tried to deal with your upset child.

Next, for the Action part you took two steps: first, you punished the behavior you didn't want. You told your child how you felt and you used time out and, perhaps, sitting in the corner for 4 minutes to demonstrate what you didn't like. You may have also practiced what you didn't like by telling your child to throw the tantrum. (Oh, I know, you have all these concerns about mixed messages. Your child knows about humor and when you mean business and when you don't. The message is always the same: "I love you and I want you to be successful in life." There's nothing mixed about that.)

Second, you taught the behavior you *do* want. You want your child to ask for help and to be cooperative.

Third, you asked your child how she feels and you demonstrated how you feel, too, when things don't go your way. You didn't focus on the anger. You focused on the relationship between the two of you. The feelings behind the anger were acknowledged and brought out into the open.

Finally, you gave your child a new way to think about being asked to pick up toys and go to bed. You are creating a new Self Statement. Your child can learn that asking for help when he or she is tired is a better way to solve a problem (handle an Event) than deciding "I must have my way all the time," which is probably what a young child is thinking when he or she is told to do something unpleasant.

You also will have given your child the opportunity to have the Four Basic Psychological Needs met. Belonging, because the two of you worked on the problem together; Power, your child influenced how you feel (but you didn't do or say things that were mean or angry); Freedom, the two of you found a better way to solve the problem; and, finally, Fun, as you hugged and praised the attempt your child made to behave as you wanted.

Helping an angry child is not easy, but, at the same time, it doesn't have to be complicated. Keep in mind that your values are more important and what and how you teach them, in the long run is more important than solving an immediate problem.

Also keep in mind that *you* are the person who decides what values are important. You need to be the powerful person in your family, not your child. Children learn how to be personally powerful by living in a safe environment with predictable consequences and rewards. The more consistent you are on living and insisting on your values, the more your child will learn self control and self esteem. Children know when their parents have their children's best interest at heart. They also know when parents are selfish and self-serving. If you deal with your child to improve his or her success in life, your child is very likely to turn out well. If you deal with your child to improve how successful you appear to your peers, friends, authority figures and the like, the less likely your child will turn out well. Managing an angry child means managing yourself first, so your goal of raising a successful adult remains clear.

WAYS TO BE ANGRY WORKSHEET

On this worksheet, list five acceptable ways for your child to let you know he or she is angry:

1. _____

2. _____

3. _____

4. _____

5. _____

Now list ways to approve of your child when he or she acts angry in the way you approve:

• _____

• _____

• _____

• _____

• _____

Now list ways you will disapprove if your child acts out in anger:

• _____

• _____

• _____

• _____

• _____

CHAPTER 11

MIX THE INGREDIENTS...

If this were a recipe book this would be the part where we put all the things in the recipe together and toss it in the oven to bake. Now, admittedly, some of my ideas may have seemed half-baked to you but I think you'll find the model we have been putting together will turn out nicely, after all.

One of the most distressing things I find, as a counselor, is that sometimes people will take ideas out of my office with a thousand good intentions and never make a commitment to actually making them a part of their life. Good ideas, unused, are no better than bad ideas. This book was written with the intent of making it easy to take a step at a time as a parent, and I hope you have done as I have suggested.

This chapter is really about looking at the ideas and putting them to use in everyday situations with your Firespitter.

In Chapter 1 we talked about putting on the oxygen mask of self control. The idea is that to be a successful parent it is important to stay *Internally Controlled.* It is crucial that you live your life according to your own values and beliefs and that you teach those beliefs and values to your child. It's also important that you realize your child will do and say things that you'll find upsetting and that is a normal part of life. Take a deep breath, slow down and remember, you are the one who controls your thoughts and feelings. If you give that control away to your child, you are no longer the one who is in control of yourself or your family.

In Chapter 2 we talked about how important it is to make sure the feelings your child feels around you are the feelings you want him or her to feel. We talked about how commercials consciously sell a feeling along with their product so that when you or I have a feeling we'll think of their product or when we want a feeling we'll think of their product.

It is the same for parenting. If you consistently "sell" the feeling of comfort and caring to your child, when he or she wants comfort and care you will be the one who is thought of. If you consistently "sell" the feeling of patience or kindness to your child, that is how you will be remembered long after the problem or experience is forgotten.   However, feelings we want others to feel mean we have to actively and purposely make those feelings a part of our life and a part of what we are trying to accomplish in every interaction.

So, first we take back our self control and then we decide what feeling is the most important one we want our child to feel when we deal with him or her.

In Chapter 3 we talked about stress and how it can make us "regress" (or go back to earlier times to solve problems). One suggestion I have is, when you find yourself becoming stressed about your child's behavior, *put your hands on your face.* Under stress our capillaries constrict and our blood moves away from our hands, feet, and skin (not to mention our Thinking brain). We often find our hands, feet, ears and even skin feels colder and perhaps clammy. When we are angry our capillaries constrict all over our body, *except our hands.* When we are angry, blood actually flows to our hands. If you find your stress is increasing and you put your hands to your face and they feel cold, you are probably experiencing stress. If you put your hands to your face and they feel warm, you are probably angry and this is *not* a good time to deal with your child. You'll need to calm down first, otherwise you may act in anger which in turn will produce fear, not learning, in your child.

However, it's important, as a parent, to have some good self-care routines. You and I need to walk, talk to friends, surround ourselves with spiritual experiences, learn some new things and continue to develop insight about ourselves. If we don't, the stress can sneak up on us and we will make decisions that we may regret later.

In Chapter Four we talked about your child's stress and how important it is to keep in mind that the *symptoms* of stress are not the *sources* of stress. There is a chart in that chapter to use to track your child's stresses over a week and a number of lists of things to look for as sources and symptoms of stress.

Chapter Five covered the four basic psychological needs we all have: Belonging, Power, Freedom and Fun. Remember how important it is to meet those needs in sequence, beginning with Belonging. Looking at your child, touching your child, telling your child how he affects you, giving your child choices and having fun are all crucial to the development of his or her self esteem.

Chapter Six is all about the three brain model we use to teach and discipline children. In that chapter we talked about how we learn first with the Survival brain, then the Emotional brain and finally the Thinking brain. The Survival brain needs rules, traditions, predictability and safety. The Emotional brain needs to know it is having an affect on others, to have strong feelings and relationships. The Emotional brain is the gateway to creative problem solving. The Thinking brain needs novelty, stimulation, challenge and the chance to solve problems. The three brains work together to solve problems, while stress tends to make us less creative, less willing to be involved in relationships, and more likely to respond in ways we learned in our childhood.

Chapter Seven is all about discipline and how important it is for us to use discipline as a way to make our children followers of our values and beliefs. We talked about the goal of raising a child who is *self-disciplined* and how angry parents often teach a child to fear but not necessarily how to change or solve problems. We are raising adults, not children, and it is more important to have a self-controlled, self-disciplined, successful adult later than a child who is always in our control today.

Chapter Eight is about taking a break. Enjoy your child. He or she is a unique creation, with wonderful skills, talents and abilities. Catch him sleeping, catch her playing, watch him at school and enjoy her for who she is whenever you can. Life is more than parenting.

Chapter Nine is all about anger and the developmental stages your child (and you and I and everyone) is going through. Remember that anger is driven by feelings and statements about the events in our lives. Anger is a motivating emotion to help us change the things we don't like. It is also possible to change our anger by changing how we talk to ourselves about life. We have as much control over anger as we do over any of our other feelings.

Chapter Ten is all about how to deal with an angry child. We talked about how important it is to work on *teaching* when a child is angry, not just on control. On the other hand, it is also important to remember that no one is perfect, including you and me and now and then the lessons are not going to get taught nearly as well as we would like to have taught them. It is important for you to decide in advance what lesson you want to teach, and then teach it on purpose.

We have talked about so many things, from diet to discipline; from a three brain model to four basic psychological needs; from stress to anger and rage. Parenting is a little like trying to fix your golf swing, it can be broken down into so many separate parts that, pretty soon, nothing seems to go right.

Always begin by observing. Observe your child, make notes, take pictures, video tape behavior, keep a journal and look for patterns that lead up to the difficult behavior. At the same time, observe yourself. What are the things that bother you the most? Are they things you think will damage your child if they continue into adulthood or are they behaviors that make you crazy because they remind you of yourself or others with whom you've had some unpleasant memories?

As a therapist, it is not unusual to find the issues a parent believes are important in their child's life are the issues the parent struggled with as a child or teenager. The concept of *projection* has been around psychology for a long time. It means we project onto others our unpleasant thoughts or feelings and then try to change them to make ourselves feel better. Our children are so much a part of ourselves, it is easy to imagine that they will struggle with the very same issues with which we struggled as children or teens. However, your child (and mine) is a uniquely created individual. It pays to keep that in mind and ask yourself, "Is this my problem or is this really a problem that belongs to my child?" Sometimes you'll find it is much more your problem than your child's. If you have had serious problems of your own growing up, if you have experienced abuse or neglect, if you have struggled with difficult habits or addictions, if you have experienced heart-wrenching defeats, then it is important that you understand the effect of these experiences on you before you decide your child is also experiencing the same problems. Sometimes the best thing for a child is to have his or her parent go to therapy for themselves before deciding the child has a serious problem.

One last little piece of advice: if your relationship with your husband or wife is under stress or is not going well, don't be surprised to find your child acting out. Children are often barometers of how well their parents' relationship is going. Remember, your child has studied every little thing about you. She can mimic your walk, your talk, your laugh and your manners. He is not insulated from the emotional upsets you face and, if he can't find the words to speak, he often will then behave badly in order to express how he feels about how you feel. Sometimes, children have been known to act badly to take the pressure off of their parents' relationship, "Mom and Dad are fighting so I will act up and they can focus on me and not on each other." I know that seems silly or even impossible, that a child would sacrifice himself for his parents, but I have seen it more than once and, when the parents' relationship improved, amazingly, the child's behavior also improved.

So, to paraphrase Robert Fulghum (<u>Everything I Ever Needed To Know I Learned In Kindergarten</u>), remember the first and most important words in the Dick and Jane readers: "Look." Or, to quote from Stephen Covey, "Seek first to understand, then be understood." Or, to go back to the beginning, "Put the oxygen mask on yourself first, before you try to help your child."

Children do come with instructions. They are self contained. If you can get to know your child well enough, the instructions will appear, right before your very eyes.

SOME FINAL THOUGHTS

This is the last worksheet in the book. Thank you for participating and for working so hard. One of the things that makes learning effective is teaching what you know to someone else. This book has been all about teaching your values and beliefs to your difficult child. However, it can also be helpful to share what you've learned with someone else.

List three things that you learned in this experience that you think you could share with someone who is struggling with their Firespitter:

1. _____

2. _____

3. _____

List three things you learned about yourself during this experience:

1. _____

2. _____

3. _____

If there is something you'd like to share with me, here is the easiest way to reach me: WEBSITE: firespitters.com

Thank you for taking the time and energy to do this work. I hope you found it helpful.

SELECTED BIBLIOGRAPHY

Ames, Gillespie, Haines, Ilg; <u>The Gesell Institute's Child from One to Six</u>; Harper & Row, New York

Armstrong, Thomas; <u>7 Kinds of Smart</u>; Penguin Books, New York

Brown, Margaret Wise, <u>The Runaway Bunny</u>; Harper & Row; New York

Braley, James M.D.; <u>Food Allergy and Nutrition Revolution</u>; New Canaan, Conn. Keats Publishing Company, 1992

Cline, Foster & Fay, Jim; <u>Parenting With Love and Logic</u>; Pinion Press; Colorado Springs, Colorado

Covey, Stephen; <u>The 7 Habits of Highly Effective People</u>; Simon and Schuster, New York

Crabb, Larry; <u>Inside Out</u>; Navpress, Boulder, Colorado

Crary, Elizabeth; <u>I'm Frustrated</u>; Parenting Press, Seattle, Washington

Crary, Elizabeth; <u>I'm Mad</u>; Parenting Press, Seattle, Washington

Crary, Elizabeth; <u>Without Spanking or Spoiling</u>; Parenting Press, Seattle, Washington

Dawson, Geraldine (ed.); <u>Autism, Nature, Diagnosis and Treatment</u>; The Guilford Press, New York, 1987; specifically chapter 15

Depree, Max; <u>Leadership Jazz</u>; Bantam Doubleday Dell Publishing Group, New York

<u>Developmental Psychology Today</u>; Crim Books, Del Mar, California

Donnellan, Anne and Paul, Rhea (eds.); <u>Handbook of Autism and Pervasive Developmental Disorders</u>; John Wiley & Sons, New York, 1987

Eastman, Meg; <u>Taming The Dragon In Your Child</u>; John Wiley & Sons, New York

Foster, Carolyn; <u>The Family Patterns Workbook</u>; Putnam Publishing Group, New York

Fruedenberger, Herbert & North, Gail; <u>Women's Burnout</u>; Doubleday Co.; Garden City, New York

Fulghum, Robert; <u>All I Really Needed To Know I Learned In Kindergarten</u>; Ivy Books, New York

Gordon, Thomas; <u>Teaching Children Self-Discipline</u>; Random House Inc.; Times Books, New York

Gordon, Thomas; <u>Discipline That Works</u>; Penguin Books, New York

Kelleher, Carol; *Triune Brain*; paper presented at Family Services America bi-annual conference, Cincinatti, Ohio

Kreidler, William; <u>Creative Conflict Resolution</u>; Scott, Foresman & Co.; Glenview, Illinois

Leman, Kevin; <u>The Birth Order Book</u>; F.H. Revell; Old Tappan, New Jersey

Marshall, James; <u>The Devil in the Classroom</u>; Schocken Books, New York

Parens, Henri, <u>Aggression In Our Children</u>; Jason Aronson Inc., Northvale, New Jersey

Triad, Paul; <u>Conversations with Preschool Children</u>; W. W. Norton & Co., New York

Weber, Rosalind; <u>Color Me Safe</u>; Weble Publishing Co.; Portland, OR.

Williams, Donna; <u>Nobody, Nowhere</u>; Times Books, New York, 1991

Windell, James; <u>8 Weeks to a Well-Behaved Child</u>; Macmillan Publishing Co.; New York

ISBN 141202044-1

9 781412 020442